The Mystery in the Room:

A Physician's Journey Treating Patients with Rare Diseases

Dr. Chuck Radis

eBook published by: Kindle Direct Publishing
Softcover: Sakamo Press

ISBN: 979-8-9999095-0-3

Cover photo: James McCarthy

Foreword

It is both a joy and privilege to be asked to write the foreword for *The Mystery in the Room,* a book that vividly captures the real-world challenges—and quiet victories and defeats—faced by both doctor and patient in the realm of complex rheumatic diseases. This is not merely a book about arthritis or rare autoimmune conditions, though it is indeed filled with fascinating and perplexing medical cases. It is, more than anything, a book about people—and about the doctor who never stopped trying to understand them.

Dr. Chuck Radis has given us a gift: stories from the frontlines of medicine, told not from the head of the exam table, but from the heart. I first came to know Dr. Radis through his case-based essays published in a professional journal for rheumatologists, and they were terrific. He has melded these and many other stories into a book that speaks to all of us—as patients, as caregivers, and as human beings—viewed and beautifully described from the other side of the bed rail.

Before he became a rheumatologist, Dr. Radis was a primary care physician on the Casco Bay Islands in Maine, a waterman and adventurer—a man who learned to listen to the wind and the waves. Later, he brought that same attentiveness to his patients. That spirit is the heartbeat of this book. Some stories unfold like gripping medical mysteries; others are deeply human narratives that remind us that even when the diagnosis is clear, the path forward can be fraught with emotional and ethical complexity.

As a rheumatologist who has practiced for over 40 years, I know the feeling when a patient and I are not in agreement—when their health belief and desired therapies diverge from what I believe they need. These moments, and many more, are poignantly and honestly portrayed throughout the book. Dr. Radis also reflects candidly on the vulnerability of caregivers and the inevitability of mistakes. *The Mystery in the Room* embodies the human values essential to both care and caring: the importance of curiosity and wonder in solving difficult medical problems, and the necessity of empathy—genuine, felt empathy—in every patient interaction. It demonstrates what I like to call "office wisdom." Whether you are a patient (as we all are at some point), or a healthcare professional seeking insight into how science and humanism must come together in the care of the sick, you will find this book both moving and illuminating.

Leonard Calabrese, DO
Professor of Medicine
Cleveland Clinic Lerner College of Medicine
Richard Fasenmeyer Chair of Clinical Immunology
Theodore F. Classen Chair of Osteopathic Research and Education, Cleveland Clinic

Introduction

The Mystery in the Room is first and foremost not a treatise on how to diagnose and treat patients with rare disorders. It is, instead, a reflection on the dance practitioners and their patients engage in as they navigate uncertainty. Arriving at a specific diagnosis in uncommon diseases takes time, persistence, and may require referrals to multiple specialists.

Because nearly all immunologic disorders are lifelong, *The Mystery in the Room* also focuses on how patients adjust (or do not adjust) to living with a chronic illness. Early on, uncertainty, anger, and denial are often present at my office visits. Over time, as the doctor/patient relationship deepens, my goal is to replace fear and anxiety with trust and understanding. I do not always meet this goal.

Many of my patients reappear in later chapters. Even without a cure, they are living their best lived lives. There are also patients who struggle with medication side effects, chronic pain, or the relentless progression of their disease. It is to these patients, in particular, that I dedicate this book.

Treatment options for rare diseases are expanding rapidly, but for those who continue to suffer, Abraham Verghese MD noted: "Healing is impossible without trust. With trust, if you can't cure, you may still heal." The founder of the osteopathic profession, A.T. Still, DO, stated that "to find health should be the object of every doctor. Anyone can find disease." A diagnosis is only the beginning. The dance goes on.

Chuck Radis, DO

Chapter 1

"In medicine, uncertainty is the water we swim in."
Dr. Lisa Sanders: *Every Patient Tells a Story: Medical Mysteries and the Art of Diagnosis*

The ER nurse, followed by the phlebotomist, followed by a medical student, flowed into Amanda's cubicle. Dr. John Benner pulled up a chair to review the case with me at the nursing station. "Here's what we got. Twelve-year-old girl with a one-week history of diffuse aches and pains, fever, and chest pain. Dad carried her in from the car. She's short of breath and requiring supplemental oxygen. Hey, thanks for coming down, I heard you were in-house. Your tie, it's got an ugly spot on it."

Dr. Benner silently handed me an alcohol swab. I looked down at an unidentifiable brown smudge on my faded tartan tie and tucked in my shirt. My stethoscope was stuffed into the back pocket of my corduroys. I do not own a white coat or a pair of surgical scrubs. During a recent weeklong backpacking trip on the Appalachian Trail in western Maine, a scraggly, snow-white beard had emerged.

"Tough exam," Dr. Benner continued. "She cried everywhere I touched her. Anyway, her breath sounds are diminished in the right lung base, could be some fluid there, we're getting a chest X-ray. She has a rash on the lower legs and her face and chest are flushed as well." He paused. "Maybe one of your diseases? Nice beard. Looks like you could pass for your wife's father."

I didn't have enough data to comment. Around us, controlled chaos; my community hospital ER hummed with activity. Remembering the alcohol swab, I opened the package and succeeded in smearing the stain further. Then I glanced at my reflection in a mirror above the sink. Wife's father? I pulled out my weekly planner from my shirt pocket and scribbled: *Shave beard tonight.*

Amanda's nurse flung open the ringed curtain and reached for an IV bag off a nearby supply cart. I cupped my hands so that she could hear me above the din. "Grab two red top tubes for me, will you? We don't want to draw her twice. I'll enter the orders in the computer. Thanks."

The nurse scowled at me but reached back for the extra red-top tubes. I focused my attention on Amanda, her rapid, shallow breathing punctuated by fitful whimpering. Instead of a hospital gown, she wore loose-fitting pink-flowered pajamas. On her feet, floppy white slippers. Her mom—they shared the same hazel-colored bob—hovered over her daughter's shoulder, whispering in her ear. When the nurse released a lever on Amanda's stretcher for the blood draw, Amanda shrieked and flailed to remain upright as if lying down was akin to drowning. I glanced at my watch and silently counted her respiratory rate. Way too high. Pain? Anxiety?

"Welcome to my world," Dr. Benner deadpanned. The nurse emerged seconds later with a fistful of blood-filled tubes. Dr. Benner handed me the chart. "Okay, your turn."

I remained seated. "No, she's short of breath. Let's get a chest X-ray first. Radiology can be processing the film while I examine Amanda and talk with her parents." A whiff of uncertainty flowed over me. Amanda was considerably younger than my average patient. As an adult rheumatologist, I'm well aware that of the more than 100 immunologic disorders rheumatologists treat, some occur only in childhood or present with different signs and symptoms than in adults. Certain drugs are approved in adults but not in children. That's why I traditionally have had a low threshold for sending complex pediatric cases two hours south to Boston's Children's Hospital.

For now though, Amanda was my responsibility. I waited, tapping out a paradiddle with my index fingers while keeping time with my right foot, a habit which emerges at times of uncertainty or stress. I had a few minutes.

Looking up from Amanda's chart, I recognized most of the nurses and support staff, including the security guard who waved me in despite the absence of an ID badge. This is my home hospital, the training site for my internship and internal medicine residency. One floor above us, my wife Sandi gave birth to Kate, now age 10, and Molly, age 7. Heck, in past years, I even moonlighted here, pulling an occasional shift for Dr. Benner.

After the X-ray technician exited the room, I pulled back the curtain, and shook hands with Amanda's dad. The mother's hand never left her daughter's shoulder. "Hi Amanda," I smiled. "Until a week ago, I understand you were okay. Are you in middle school?" Sometimes 12-year-olds can be quite chatty. Instead, she locked eyes with her mom.

As we talked, I gently examined Amanda's hands. Why the hands? They're innocent to touch yet sometimes hold the key to diagnosis. The fingers were stone cold, the knuckles slightly swollen and tender. Beneath several nails, a thin black streak, a nail infarct, was clearly evident. Internally I grimaced. Nail infarcts are a subtle sign of damage to the smallest blood vessels. They are often seen with serious infections…but can also be observed in several rare immunologic diseases. Did Amanda have a life-threatening infection? I glanced down at the order sheet and noted that Dr. Benner had ordered urine and blood cultures to rule this out. Good.

I consciously kept my voice soft and unhurried, and asked Amanda's mother, "What was the first thing you noticed out of the ordinary with your daughter?"

"Two weeks ago, the fevers started up. Every night, just over one hundred degrees, then the muscle aching and joint pain. I've kept her home the last four days and treated the fever and pain with Tylenol. She's up off and on all night lately trying to sleep propped up with three or even four pillows."

"I think it goes back farther than that." Amanda's dad, who had been leaning against the sink, took a seat on the other side of the stretcher. "Remember the rash last month after she spent the day at Funtown on the water slides? It looked different than a sunburn, you know, not red all over, kind of blotchy, and that was the first time her muscles ached. I thought she had some kind of bug."

As he spoke, I methodically continued my exam. Inside Amanda's mouth I identified two large ulcers on the edge of her tongue. Pulling back a swatch of hair, behind the right ear I discovered a bare patch of pink scalp the size of a nickel. Amanda scowled as I leaned in for a closer look. Evidently, she had also discovered the bald spot. "I hate my hair. Don't touch it."

"Sorry." Stepping back, I studied the pink rash extending across Amanda's nose and onto the cheeks, sparing the outer edges of both nostrils. Her mother rolled up her pajamas to above the knees. From the mid-calves to the ankles, the skin was peppered with angry red spots. Wrong rash for parvovirus. Wrong rash for measles or mononucleosis. This was much more worrisome.

"Just don't lie me down!" she begged in a panicked whisper. Recalling Amanda's reaction when the nurse had lain her flat, I reassured her that I could finish the examination with her sitting upright.

The din of the ER faded as I placed my stethoscope on her chest. What was it one of my former attendings preached about heart sounds? *You may think you hear with your ears, but you listen with your mind.* The human brain has an uncanny ability to isolate and interpret sounds by suppressing awareness of background noise. I closed my eyes and focused.

Initially, the only abnormal finding I heard was Amanda's racing heart. But just before I lifted my stethoscope from her chest, I detected a faint creaking, leathery sound between heart beats, a sound I hear, perhaps, once every two or three years. There it was again, the distinctive sound associated with inflammation of the sack surrounding the heart, or in medical parlance: a pericardial rub. Amanda's panic now made sense; pericardial pain dramatically worsens with lying flat.

Even more concerning, a pericardial rub is often associated with fluid around the heart, and this can be life threatening. To assess this, I wrapped a blood pressure cuff around Amanda's arm and inflated the cuff. Instead of taking a traditional blood pressure I was interested in whether the blood pressure varied as she breathed in and out. At a blood pressure of 100, I felt a pulse at the wrist, but ominously, only as she breathed out. With inspiration the pulse disappeared. Only when I reached a pressure of 86 did I detect a continuous heartbeat.

The hair on the back of my neck tingled. Breathing in and out usually has minimal effect on blood pressure readings. My simple test suggested that not only was there fluid around the heart, but that it was approaching a critical level, compressing the heart like a giant fist and dropping Amanda's blood pressure. Emerging from the exam cubicle, I spotted Dr. Benner as he reviewed Amanda's EKG. He motioned me over. "Poor kid. Look at these changes. Classic for pericarditis. Did you hear a pericardial rub?"

I chose my words carefully. "Yes, it's faint but definitely there. We need to confirm this with an ultrasound, but by my simple testing, the more immediate problem is that the amount of fluid surrounding this young lady's heart is putting her at risk of abruptly dropping her blood pressure, perhaps even dying."

Behind us, the X-ray tech hung Amanda's chest X-ray on the screen and flipped on the view box. The silhouette of the heart was dramatically enlarged, almost certainly a combination of the heart itself and the fluid surrounding it. We turned back to where we could see Amanda through the edge of the exam curtain. Amanda's blood pressure on the cardiac monitor had dropped to 90. She sat bolt upright, her breathing coming in shallow panicky gasps. No wonder the poor kid couldn't lie down, that feeling of drowning was real.

"John, there's no question that Amanda has SLE (*systemic lupus erythematosus*). Even without blood work, the butterfly facial rash, inflamed joints, patchy hair loss, and pericardial rub are all classic for the diagnosis. The fluid around her heart needs to be drained by vascular surgery as soon as possible. We need to transfer her over to Maine Medical Center, like, thirty minutes ago."

7

"Karen." Dr. Benner's voice was sharp and focused. Gone was the laid-back, you've got a stain on your tie repartee. He clicked out a series of orders. "Turn our young lady's oxygen up to six per minute in cubicle # 5. Start another IV in the opposite arm and run in a liter of normal saline over the next 15 minutes. Have the front desk contact the Buxton ambulance that left here five minutes ago and tell them to turn around. We need a transfer, now." He shot me an uncertain look. "How much steroid do you want to give her?"

"One thousand milligrams."

"Make that a thousand milligrams of Solu-Medrol. Send Tom up to pharmacy, stat. Let's get that Solu-Medrol infused before the transfer."

The laboratory technician handed me Amanda's results. More bad news. As if the fluid around her heart wasn't bad enough, the poor kid was in kidney failure and her blood counts were in the toilet. Half-closing my eyes, I reviewed where we stood, acutely aware that another team of physicians was going to assume Amanda's care in the Maine Medical Center ER, and I wanted to ensure I wasn't overlooking any critical data that required immediate attention.

I parted the curtain and taking Amanda's parents aside, briefly reviewed the diagnosis of SLE with them, and why we needed to transfer their daughter to Maine Medical Center. "We suspect that there is considerable fluid around Amanda's heart, and a surgeon will need to drain the fluid."

"Will you be on the team at Maine Medical Center?" the father asked.

"Yes. I'm on staff at both hospitals. I'll be coordinating her lupus care."

Returning to her cubicle, I realized that Amanda was drifting into the vacant, dissociated gaze that patients get just prior to losing consciousness. The blood pressure on the monitor continued to slide: 88, 86, 84. I turned up the rate of her intravenous fluids and watched the creamy steroid solution infuse into the opposite arm. The blood pressure leveled off and rose ever so slightly.

In a pinch, I'm confident that Dr. Benner is capable of sticking a large bore needle through Amanda's lower chest into the sac surrounding the heart to drain the constrictive fluid, but it's a high-risk procedure and ideally should be performed by an experienced cardiologist or vascular surgeon under ultrasound. If the needle inadvertently pricks the heart muscle it could trigger a fatal bleed. Then I patted Amanda on her forearm and told her family she was going to be okay.

Moments later, the ambulance arrived and two EMTs wheeled a stretcher into our cubicle. Dr. Benner stood by. Tucked under his arm was a procedure tray, just in case he needed to aspirate fluid from around the heart. We watched silently as Amanda slid onto the transfer stretcher. I instructed the ambulance attendants to avoid lying Amanda flat. Her mother never let go of her daughter's shoulder as she squeezed into the back of the ambulance.

Minutes later, at the Maine Medical Center emergency room, after an ultrasound confirmed the fluid around her heart, Amanda was whisked up to the operating room where a cardiac surgeon awaited. More than a pint of straw-colored fluid was removed from the sac around the heart, and a drain was inserted through the chest wall to prevent re-accumulation. Almost immediately, her blood pressure rebounded to 118/78; her pulse dropped to 96. The immediacy of Amanda's death was averted.

The term, lupus—derived from the Latin word for wolf—refers to the disfiguring facial rash of lupus patients. And while it's true that some lupus patients have a disfiguring lupus rash suggestive of a predator's bite, there are many patients in whom the skin is entirely spared. The variability of the disease is breathtaking. The diagnosis may be readily apparent, as it was in Amanda that day, or elude diagnosis for years. In medical school, I was taught that lupus and syphilis were the Great Imposters, meaning their signs and symptoms mimic a host of more common disorders. On medical rounds, it was always a safe bet to include lupus in any perplexing case.

In contrast to another immunologic disorder, rheumatoid arthritis, where the joints are the primary target, widespread organ inflammation is the rule in lupus. The lungs, heart, blood, skin, kidneys, liver, eyes, and central nervous system may all be targeted simultaneously in a critically ill patient, or the disease may unfold over months or years in those with smoldering disease.

But what exactly is lupus? As a classic autoimmune disease, it is a case of mistaken identity writ large. The immune system in patients like Amanda is in chronic overdrive, effectively performing its primary job—protecting the body from infection—while triggering inflammation and damage in normal tissues. On laboratory testing, ninety-nine percent of lupus patients develop anti-nuclear antibodies (ANA). Many patients have additional antibodies to proteins found within the nucleus of cells; the list is long and growing.

The exact sequence of events leading to lupus is unclear, but like many immunologic disorders, the disease has both a genetic predisposition and suspected environmental, hormonal, and infectious triggers. Although men may develop lupus, it is primarily a disease of women.

The next morning, I stopped by Maine Medical Center before office hours and recommended two more days of high-dose steroids for Amanda. The surgery team assessed the chest wound where pericardial fluid drained through a tube to a bedside collecting system. Hematology consulted on the severe anemia and low platelet counts. A nephrologist recommended a kidney biopsy.

As she ate breakfast on her third day in the intensive care unit, Amanda's eyes suddenly rolled back and she suffered a seizure—a known complication of lupus. The force of the seizure ripped the IV from her forearm, splattering blood and IV fluid onto the bedsheet and floor. The oxygen line snapped off the wall mount and Amanda's oxygen level plummeted. Fortunately, the catheter extending through her chest wall draining the fluid from around her heart was pinned to her hospital gown and remained in place.

Within minutes, a tube was placed in Amanda's windpipe and she was placed on a ventilator. A chest X-ray confirmed the worst; during the seizure she'd aspirated a portion of her breakfast. A scan of the brain, thankfully, didn't demonstrate a stroke or bleed. A neurologist performed a spinal tap and the results were consistent with central nervous system inflammation from lupus. As the days dragged by, only her youth saved her. High-dose steroids were critically necessary in her treatment but increased the likelihood of a resistant infection. Thankfully, by day six Amanda was off the ventilator.

That morning, I wrote an extended chart note, knowing from previous experience that while each medical specialty has a "piece" of lupus, my training as a rheumatologist and my years spent in primary care would help me see the patient beyond the confines of a single organ system. I knew that after the pericarditis resolved and the chest drain was pulled, Amanda would not need to see a vascular surgeon. As her blood counts rebounded, hematology follow-up might be unnecessary. The neurologist who performed the spinal tap and prescribed her seizure medications would continue to see her as an outpatient, but the focus would be narrow. Nephrology follow-up would be critical, but the immune-suppressive medications would overlap considerably with rheumatology.

Rheumatologists see their lupus patients for decades, through periods of remission and relapse, blending medications according to disease activity, striving to control the disease without over-suppressing the immune system. I liken my job as a rheumatologist to adjusting the damper in a fireplace: an open damper allows the fire of uncontrolled lupus to run rampant through the body. Close the damper too tightly and the immune system is smothered and infections occur frequently. Using a combination of medications, I aim for an even flame, a competent immune system. It can be a tough balance to maintain.

But how *does* one manage lupus? There is no simple recipe. For mild disease, and there are many patients with mild disease, minimizing sun exposure--a potential trigger for flares—is critically important. Sunblock, sun-protective clothing, and minimizing outdoor activities on bright sunny days is recommended. For active skin disease or inflammatory arthritis, hydroxychloroquine (Plaquenil) is frequently prescribed.

Plaquenil has a fascinating backstory. Bark from the Peruvian "fever tree," *Cinchona officinalis,* was imported to Europe in the 1600's as a treatment for malaria. During World War II, quinine, a synthetic derivative of the bark, was prescribed to as many as three million Allied soldiers to prevent malaria in the South Pacific. And while quinine proved to be an effective medication to prevent malaria, soldiers with pre-existing lupus or rheumatoid arthritis were surprised that their symptoms improved as well. A decade after the war, Plaquenil, a synthetic descendent of the Peruvian "fever tree," was approved for the long-term management of lupus. Michelle Petri, MD, the director of the Lupus Center at Johns Hopkins University School of Medicine, has said, "It is the only medicine we have that has been proven in multiple studies to improve lupus survival."

Unfortunately, while Plaquenil is effective in mild lupus, it cannot control severe lupus inflammation. In these patients, prednisone is often prescribed. Acting like a wet blanket on the immune system (closing the damper), prednisone blocks the production of multiple inflammatory proteins. Given in massive doses, prednisone (or the intravenous formulation Amanda received, Solu-Medrol) acts quickly, and if an injured organ has a wisp of function remaining, the drug may stave off organ failure. All too often though, side effects soon emerge and office visits become a war of wills. My patients want less but the disease often demands more.

Amanda needed a second medication, a slower acting, powerful immune-suppressant that could gradually allow us to taper prednisone. After lunch, the nephrologist and I met with Amanda's parents to discuss the results of her kidney biopsy. The nephrologist explained that just as rapidly dividing cancer cells can be eliminated by chemotherapy, the immune system cells responsible for Amanda's lupus kidney damage are also treated with chemotherapy. We both recommended six monthly infusions of a medication called Cytoxan.

"What's more," I added, "At the same time, we'll use another medication to shield the ovaries from the side effects of these medications to preserve fertility. As sick as Amanda is, we believe that she will recover, and in future years she'll have the option of having children."

After a few minutes, Amanda's shell-shocked parents gave their consent. A week later, her kidney function showed signs of improvement and Amanda was off supplemental oxygen. The constricting pain of her heart inflammation and the tortuous aching in her muscles and joints had resolved. At twelve years old, she was discharged on a smorgasbord of six medications.

Through her high school years, Amanda's care remained a challenge. At one point, she was a no-show at four consecutive office visits. Her parents separated and subsequently divorced. She became depressed and our visits were often adversarial. In the summer between her junior and senior years she stopped all of her medications, and following a night of binge drinking, suffered another seizure and was admitted to Maine Medical Center in kidney failure. This triggered another six-month course of chemotherapy and high-dose steroids. Miraculously, the disease was beaten back and she avoided dialysis.

Then, shortly before her senior prom, Amanda decided to go with a friend to a tanning booth with predictable results; the ultraviolet light triggered a lupus rash and dozens of blisters erupted over her upper chest and face. The open sores became infected and, a few days later, she was found by her father unconscious on the kitchen floor with a life-threatening infection.

Miraculously, she survived.

Her parents (who, after their divorce lived around the block from each other) stepped up and insisted on counseling for Amanda and alternated weeks driving her to doctors appointments and therapy sessions. Her disease stabilized. After graduating from high school, Amanda volunteered at a local veterinarian clinic and picked up a part-time job at a nearby McDonald's. Over time, she stuck with her medications, even the prednisone, which she hated more than anything. Slowly, her disease came under long-term control.

Six years after she was first hospitalized, I noticed Amanda's name on my list of morning patients. She was early. That could be good, I thought, or it could be bad. Be sharp. I walked by her exam room and peeked through the partially open door: *no facial rash, looks comfortable, appears upbeat,* and raised an eyebrow. *There's nothing wrong with a nose ring*. I asked my nurse, Joanne, to send her down for routine laboratory studies.

I returned to my office and opened up a bag of Fritos. Joanne knocked on the door. "Heads up; Amanda is wondering if you're going to stop the prednisone." I rubbed my forehead. *Maybe.* A few minutes later, the question hung in the background as I sat down across from Amanda and opened her chart. In addition to the nose ring, she sported a hummingbird tattoo on her forearm and a flower tattoo above her right ankle. She picked up a magazine, opened it, shut it, and slumped deeper into her chair.

I asked, "Did the hair regrow above the right ear where I injected the bare spot with cortisone last visit?" Without a word, Amanda pulled back a lock of hair. The scalp had filled in with normal appearing hair. "Good. How's school?"

"I'm taking a class at the community college in psychology. It's okay, I mean I don't need a psychology class to tell me that I'm whacked, but it's...interesting. I got a B plus on the first test."

"That's great. Hey! Congratulations! Are you still volunteering at the veterinarian clinic?"

"The vet is paying me. I mean, minimum wage, but I'm making some money for fun stuff. He's awesome." Twirling a pen, she pointed to my feet. "Your socks, they don't match. Not even close. How'd you get that hole in the cuff of your pants?"

I glanced down to confirm her observation. "Thanks for noticing." Then I methodically continued my exam. There were no oral ulcers or facial rash. The lungs and heart were normal. None of her joints were swollen or tender.

Her exam was, well, normal.

Amanda straightened up in her chair. "Lupus sucks. It sucked when I was twelve and it sucks now and it'll suck when—and if—I make it to thirty. But you know, I'm okay with that. My counselor says that I'm doing a better job of…get this, 'living in the present.' Brilliant. So…what do you think?" she asked. "Can I stop the prednisone?"

For a moment, we sat in silence. Over the years, there had been so many flares, so many relapses. Honestly, the thought of stopping the last miniscule dose of prednisone scared the hell out of me. The laboratory tech knocked on the door with Amanda's results. After reviewing the numbers, I handed the paper to Amanda, who was by now an old hand at interpreting her blood counts and kidney tests. Except for mild permanent kidney damage, the results were essentially normal. With significant trepidation, I recommended that she stop the last 2.5 mg of prednisone.

Not that she was cured. In her purse a pillbox contained medications to control the collateral damage she'd suffered from lupus: hypertension, elevated cholesterol, anxiety, depression. And of course, she remained on Plaquenil, her best hope for remaining in remission. I think she finally understood this.

The visit over, I stood and shook her hand. "The tiny dose of prednisone we're discontinuing may turn out to be important," I cautioned her. "Please call the office if you feel your lupus is heading in the wrong direction. Otherwise, I'll see you back here in two months."

I turned to go and Amanda impulsively reached over and playfully punched me in the shoulder. "Yes!" she shouted, and skipped down the hall.

Chapter 2

"If we don't change the direction we're headed, we'll end up where we are going."
Chinese proverb

It was never my goal to become a doctor. My droopy-eyed, disengaged family doctor wore tailored suits that looked like he'd slept in them. When he leaned his belly against my side and peered into my ears with his otoscope, his breath was an admixture of Listerine and Marlboros. Once, I caught him surreptitiously peek at my name on the chart as he entered the exam room and, without raising his eyes, ask, "And how are you today, my good friend…Chuck."

As a 10-year-old I knew with absolute certainty: I was not his good friend Chuck.

Having now practiced medicine for nearly 40 years, if I met him today, I would be less judgmental and more sympathetic. He might be a colleague or friend. Who knows what losses he'd endured over his practice life? Was he depressed? Divorced? Estranged from his children? Had the pressures of caring for his patients, the endless nights on call, led him to alcoholism or drug addiction? Was he getting help?

Though I grew up in suburban Cranford, New Jersey, only thirty minutes from New York City, I fished for trout in the local river. My early connection to fishing and the outdoors was a lasting gift from both my mother Shirley—who was raised on a farm in West Virginia without indoor plumbing, and my father Frank—the hard-working son of Italian immigrants, and the first in his family to graduate from college. Early in their marriage they had lived in Henderson, Nevada, where my brothers, Rick and Steve and I were born. A dog-eared photo I keep of them on the bank of the nearby Colorado River shows them proudly holding a brace of dripping trout.

My father's work as a chemical engineer brought the family east to New Jersey where he managed a plant which manufactured DDT for the Montrose Chemical Company. "Manufactured DDT" is a bland description for a plant which spewed out billowing, sulfurous emissions into the atmosphere 24-7, 365 days a year. When he returned home each evening, no matter how much he scrubbed, the odor remained a part of him. And he was not embarrassed or ashamed of this. Like many of his generation, he believed that science held the answers to some of society's most vexing public health problems. And it was beyond dispute that in Africa, wherever DDT was sprayed and mosquito populations plummeted, the number of malaria and yellow fever cases dropped sharply.

In 1962, Rachael Carson's book, *Silent Spring*, linked DDT exposure to steep declines in bird populations, and triggered a national debate over the environmental safety of the widely used insecticide. Although Carson did not cite studies demonstrating health risks in humans, she recommended vigorous research to investigate this possibility.

In response (I later learned), my father, who by then headed Montrose Chemical in New Jersey, was asked by the chemical industry to debate Carson on CBS national TV. I would imagine that he was picked, in part, because he radiated an easy-going sincerity, a man who could reassure the public that the use of DDT was both safe and effective. In the minds of most scientists, himself included, there was no question, DDT saved lives.

Even so, he wanted to read *Silent Spring* before agreeing to the debate. Each night, bone tired after another long day at work, he cracked open *Silent Spring* and reviewed the science behind Carson's claims. In those days, fact-checking was not a simple matter. He may have relied on his old chemistry textbooks, or checked books out of the library. Perhaps he called a former professor at Case Western University, where he obtained his chemical engineering degree. It was slow, tedious work. By the time he finished *Silent Spring*, my father was shaken to the core. He informed his superiors that based on the data Carson presented he agreed with her conclusions. This was a serious, well-researched book.

The "CBS Reports" debate went on, but another chemist represented the chemical industry. The contrast between Carson in her rocking chair on the porch of her Maine cottage and the industry spokesperson could not have been more striking. The chemist wore a white lab coat and tie, and stood in front of beakers and Bunsen burners. He seemed to talk down to Carson, even belittle her. The debate forever changed the public's perception of pesticides. The use of DDT was banned in the United States in 1972.

The stress and long hours of my father's job left little time for family. Even when he was home, he was frequently called in the middle of the night, problem-solving through stuck valves and dangerously high tank pressures at his chemical plant. Under the constant stress of working 60 to 80 hours per week, he developed a two-pack-a-day cigarette habit and his hair prematurely grayed and thinned. A former college wrestler, he had little time to walk or stay in shape. Two years after he turned down the debate with Rachael Carson, he arrived home, collapsed on the couch, and died from a massive heart attack.

He was 44 years old.

At the time, he was designing a DDT production plant to be built in Acapulco, Mexico. Although Rachel Carson had introduced him to the negative impacts of DDT on the environment, on balance, he continued to believe that DDT did more good than harm. He didn't live long enough to think otherwise.

My mother was left with the task of raising my two older brothers and me despite crushing depression. She returned to nursing and endured the chaos of our teenage years, our risk taking, our anger. She never remarried.

I have few memories of my father, but I do remember that he loved fishing. The year before he died, he taught me the finer points of using a fly rod and reading a stream. When I was frustrated by a "bird's nest" (a hopelessly tangled line) he patiently worked through the mess and said, "To catch a trout, you need your line in the water." It was, I like to think, his way of telling me, *when faced with a complex problem, stay calm, analyze the data, and work through the setbacks. Keep your line in the water.*

Memory is malleable. I could have focused on his inability to say no to work and say yes to his family. Instead, I choose to remember him as my mother and his friends and colleagues remembered him, a kind man who loved his work, who was just beginning to evolve a social consciousness. After he died, I fished more, not less. Even a river in the suburbs of New Jersey can be a healing elixir for a fatherless boy.

Through high school I binged on alcohol but avoided drugs, excelling in subjects I was interested in but barely paying attention in classes I was not. Sports mattered. Girls mattered. Hiking and camping mattered. For decades after my father died, I was unwilling, perhaps unable to cry. Somehow, I survived my teenage years, thanks to a close-knit group of friends and early mornings on the river.

Despite my uneven high school grades, I was accepted at Bates College in Lewiston, Maine in 1971. When I announced to my mother my inclination to delay college and work on a commercial fishing boat, her face paled. As a single mother who had suffered through the rollercoaster of raising three emotionally damaged boys, now her youngest was balking at higher education. She brought in the heavy artillery, her brother Thurmond, a Methodist minister, who lectured me on the sacrifices my mother had made, and my obligation, no, my duty, to go to college. Reluctantly, I agreed to go.

At Bates, I picked biology as a major, primarily because of my interest in anything connected to the water. A future career in marine biology vied with a dream of making a living as a professional pool player. I pursued both dreams lightly, adopting a philosophy of engaging only halfway in any activity with the motto: "Always leave yourself an out."

That is, until Professor Andy Balber addressed our class on the first day of an introductory immunology course in the fall of my sophomore year. Before Dr. Balber's class, I had dutifully attended classes and kind of, sort-of-studied for exams, but in truth, I was just doing the minimum to get by.

"As you may know," he began, "T cells [specialized white blood cells] are important regulators of the immune system. And what do we know about how T cells communicate with other cells?" The question hung over the lecture hall as he clicked to a blank slide and tapped the screen. "Nothing. Absolutely nothing." I sat up in my seat and closed my eyes, visualizing a T cell as a billiard ball, smooth as a baby's bottom, its surface markings—critical communication receptors—a complete unknown. For emphasis, Dr. Balber added, "There's a Nobel Prize awaiting the researcher who discovers how receptors on T cells contribute to the regulation of the immune system."

I was not on track to be that student.

In the following weeks, the world of immunology burst from our textbooks. He paced the lecture hall and breathlessly described the human immune system as mirroring a successful military operation, or a smoothly running complex society. It was as subtle as the overtones and counterpoints of a beautiful symphony and as overpowering as a thunderstorm. Or as one of my medical colleagues, Ed Fels, MD, later remarked: "The immune system speaks a different language…akin to a microscopic orchestra. Instead of notes the cells communicate through cytokines and other small molecular messengers."

In retrospect, it was a defining moment in my own transition from a passive, desultory student to a passionate learner. I continued playing pool late into the night, but drank less and found myself daydreaming about immunology.

The following summer, less lost, but by no means focused on a future career, I picked up a job on my hometown garbage truck. Heavy physical labor had always appealed to me and I was proud of my ability to lift and empty can after can into the compactor. In one memorable encounter, I greeted my favorite high school English teacher as I jumped off the rear of the truck and emptied his barrel of trash. Mr. Marcus nearly spilled his coffee in shock and disappointment that one of his favorite students had ended up working on a garbage truck. “Can’t beat the hours!” I yelled to him as the truck roared away.

He scrambled for a reply. “The man who is happy is fulfilling the purpose of existence.”

“Dostoevsky!” I shouted back as the truck rounded the corner.

Despite my newfound interest in immunology (and ignoring my mother’s wishes), at the end of my sophomore year, I took a leave of absence from Bates College and headed west to Oregon, where I failed to land a job on a commercial fishing boat. Undeterred, I strapped my belongings onto the rear rack of a well-used Schwinn and bicycled down the west coast of California, working long enough in a fish market in southern California to extend my trip down the spine of Baja, Mexico with my friends George and Bill.

It was in Baja where I met Dr. Dave, a family practice physician, at a local cantina in a remote mountain village. One weekend each month, he flew his Piper Cub plane from San Diego to a high-desert landing strip in the Sierra de la Giganta, where he provided prenatal care, manipulated injured backs, stitched up injuries, and managed diabetes and hypertension. He’d been doing this “gig,” as he called it, in addition to his full-time family practice in San Diego, for years. Dressed in dusty jeans and a gray T-shirt, Dr. Dave spoke fluent Spanish. Though he was clearly exhausted, we talked deep into the night about his devotion to patient care.

Dr. Dave was not an MD. He was a DO (Doctor of Osteopathic Medicine). I learned that DO's have taken a holistic approach to medical care since Andrew Still founded the first osteopathic medical school in Kirksville, Missouri in 1892. At the core of osteopathic medicine is the recognition that every organ system in the body is interconnected, and that treating the whole person is the physician's primary responsibility.

Having never met a DO, I was unaware that osteopathic medicine existed in a parallel universe to allopathic (MD) medicine. Both require four years of medical school. Both offer residencies in everything from family practice to cardiology to pediatrics to surgery. Only osteopathic medical students learn the art of manipulation as an adjunct to standard medical treatments. By morning, I knew I had found my people. I would become an osteopathic physician. And honestly, my earliest interactions with my MD family doctor, and the very fact that in some circles at the time, osteopathic physicians were looked down upon as less than equal to MD's, lent an unconscious attraction to the profession. It is not necessarily a bad thing to maintain a small chip on one's shoulder.

The chance encounter with Dr. Dave (sadly, I can't recall his name; perhaps he never told me), was akin to a spiritual transformation, a calling to patient care. Despite my less than stellar grades my first two years of college, I never doubted that I would become a physician.

Chapter 3

Not to say that the rest was easy. In my last two years at Bates College, my study habits improved and my grades took off. I worked part-time as an ambulance attendant and found that under stress, my heart rate remained slow and steady. Like my father, I could block out distractions and hyper-focus on problem solving.

In my senior year, I met with the Dean of Students at Bates and announced my intention to apply to medical school. He looked at my grades the first two years of college, and raised an eyebrow. Then he reviewed my last two years of A's. "You know Chuck," he said, patting me on the shoulder, "I've got to tell you, that ship has sailed."

Only it hadn't. I did well on the Medical College Admission Test (MCAT) and the Kansas City College of Osteopathic Medicine admitted me, I suspect, more on my trajectory and potential than my grade point average. Of course, it didn't hurt that an article I wrote on osteopathic medicine was published by a regional magazine.

Shortly after my acceptance to medical school, I met my future spouse, Sandi (who was a year behind me at Bates College), and a month later we drove to New Jersey in my dilapidated, faded red (she says pink) Toyota truck to meet my mother. The two women bonded immediately. Together, they shared a love of family, straightforward conversation, and an unshakable belief in women's and men's freedom to choose (at a time when women's liberation was ascendant, Sandi's college senior thesis was titled: *Men's Liberation*).

Although I am convinced that Sandi could have pursued a career as an airline pilot or police detective, her focus on proper parenting never wavered from when she read her first copy of *Family Circle* at age nine. As the youngest of three children, she was a precocious reader, and would circle recommendations in the magazine and pass them on to her parents at the breakfast table. When she disagreed with their decisions, she would remind them that the people who wrote for *Family Circle* were experts. *So, pay attention.* What a pain in the butt.

For my mother's part, she was an honest, liberal-minded, Methodist West Virginian. Our neighborhood in Cranford, New Jersey, was primarily Jewish and many of my close school friends were either Jewish or Black. After my father died, my mother worked the night shift as a floor nurse at a nearby hospital. One morning she joined a group of women for breakfast at the end of her shift and the conversation drifted to grievances the nurses held against Jewish patients and the Jewish medical staff. My mom listened quietly until she had finished her coffee, then picked up her tray and locked eyes with the main perpetrator in the group. "I've got to hurry and pick up my son for his Saturday morning Hebrew school class." Without another word, she left.

Although I had returned to Bates College with a passion for science following my bike trip down the Baja peninsula, in many respects I was still a work in progress. My scatterbrained behavior nearly doomed my budding relationship with Sandi. During our first visit to New Jersey, my truck ran out of gas, and we walked hand-in-hand to a nearby gas station. I pumped a gallon of gas into a container and reached into my back pocket only to find that my wallet was missing. Sandi remained at the station to ensure that I returned and paid for the gas. I drove home and discovered my wallet in a pair of pants I had draped over a chair. I was hungry so I fixed myself a sandwich and a bowl of ice cream and opened the Compton's Encyclopedia on the kitchen table. Time passed. The kitchen phone rang. It was Sandi at the gas station. What was holding me up?

I placed my half-eaten sandwich ever so slowly back on the plate and closed the encyclopedia. Did I admit to Sandi that I had completely forgotten her? Yes. And that probably saved our relationship. While Sandi offered encouragement and direction, she drew the line at micromanaging my absent-minded trail of forgotten items. Boundaries were clearly set. It was my problem, not hers.

We bonded in surprising ways. For instance, after meeting Sandi, I never again went to a barber. For nearly five decades she has trimmed my hair with her family's antique Manning and Bowman haircut kit. I dislike going to a store to purchase clothes. In fact, if it was up to me, I would never, ever shop. Sandi finds great joy in buying second hand "bargains" at Goodwill, and outfits me in a range of lightly used ties, shirts, and replacement winter gloves and hats. Between my haircut and second hand clothes, I tend towards a casual, "absent-minded professor" look, which I am absolutely comfortable with. We joke that since we've met, I have been in a form of "assisted care."

And I appreciate her idiosyncrasies. The veins on the back of Sandi's left hand spell out: HI! She almost never wears make-up, enjoys belly dancing, and recalls every verse from childhood camp songs. She was an accomplished college field hockey player and played the bassoon in the Bates College orchestra. A creature of habit, she eats the same breakfast day after day, month after month. I appreciate her tortoise-colored beret, which is fortunate, since it is the first (and only) fashion accessory she puts on each day, and the last to come off.

Her unique work resume includes a master's degree in social work and stints as a child and family therapist followed by twelve years as a plumber and electrician assistant on Peaks Island. When friends are surprised that she has worked in the trades, that she lugged heavy tools under crawl spaces and fixed clogged drains, she says, "There's actually not much difference between plumbing and family therapy. One way or the other, you deal with people's shit."

As my college graduation neared, we both dreaded the toll on our relationship if I went off to medical school in the Midwest and Sandi remained at Bates for her senior year. Was I obliged to begin medical school as soon as possible? Or was my evolving relationship with Sandi more important?

I chose Sandi, and wrote a formal letter to the dean at the medical school in Kansas City asking if I could defer my admission for a year. Awaiting his response, I worried that he would inform me it was now or never, that there were dozens of applicants who would sacrifice anything to go to medical school. Instead, he simply wrote back, "Permission granted."

That year, Sandi and I shared an apartment off-campus and I continued my part-time job as an ambulance attendant, and that fall worked as a public health immunization technician. Instead of slogging away in a laboratory to improve my science resume, I waitered at a local steak house and briefly worked with pre-school children at Head Start. Together with my previous summer jobs roofing houses and working on my hometown's garbage truck, I unknowingly was building the social skills necessary to connect with a wide spectrum of patients in a busy medical practice. After all, when a doctor makes the correct diagnosis, the job is only half-done. What follows is equally important: a clear explanation (in nonmedical terms) of what's wrong, a review of treatment options, and follow-through to ensure the plan is working.

In medical school I flourished. Sure, I continued to wear mismatched socks but my mind seemed to quietly place scientific concepts and patient information in tidy, uncluttered rooms where they could be readily recalled. I was captivated by every malady under the sun, but particularly with rare, autoimmune diseases. And like many medical students, I was influenced by the illnesses of my own extended family. Autoimmune thyroid disease had affected my mother. My oldest brother suffered from Crohn's disease, my father from psoriasis, both immune-mediated disorders. My grandfather Rice Beavers, in West Virginia, was wheelchair bound, then bedbound for the last seven years of his life from the devastating effects of rheumatoid arthritis and Parkinson's disease.

Following graduation, I began a three-year internal medicine residency at a 160-bed osteopathic hospital in Portland, Maine. My interest in rare disorders continued under the guidance of Phil Slocum, DO, the chief of the internal medicine program. Dr. Slocum taught his residents to maintain an open mind and to constantly reevaluate a diagnosis if the patient failed to improve with standard treatment. If you hear hoofbeats, perhaps it's not always a horse, it could be a zebra—a rare disease.

One night, I admitted an elderly woman from the emergency room with a low-grade fever and confusion. When I examined her, she groaned wherever she was touched. The usual approach in a disoriented, elderly patient is to assume an underlying infection is present, obtain a chest X-ray, urine and blood cultures, and begin intravenous fluids and antibiotics. I checked the usual boxes on the order sheet and was soon on to my next admission.

Several days later, our patient was no better and nothing was growing from her cultures. Infection was unlikely. Nursing informed us that our patient wasn't eating or drinking and that when she was moved, she cried out in pain. We were faced with the dilemma of placing a feeding tube to ensure she received adequate nutrition, or allowing her to die. A feeding tube was placed. She pulled it out. Gentle restraints were placed (there is no such thing as gentle restraints), and the feeding tube was reinserted.

That afternoon, the woman's niece confronted our entourage of medical students, Dr. Slocum, and me outside the patient's room. She was outraged at the sight of her aunt in restraints, and demanded we remove the feeding tube and allow the poor woman to die. We considered this, but decided to defer the decision for another 24 hours.

The next day, another niece visited, and the story could not have been more different. "Only two weeks ago, my aunt was up and about, doing her own cooking and chores. She was looking forward to flying to California next month to receive a lifetime achievement award from the National Poetry Foundation." As evidence she handed us a newspaper clipping.

Shocked (and not a little chagrined), we regarded our patient with fresh eyes. Dr. Slocum reread my admission history and physical and shook his head at its brevity and lack of depth. It was time to reassess our original diagnosis of infection. Dr. Slocum pointed to a line from my admit note, *hurts everywhere* and asked,

"Dr. Radis can you demonstrate this for us?" Reluctantly, I gently lifted an arm. The patient groaned and jerked her arm away.

Dr. Slocum leaned over and whispered in her ear, "May I examine you?" From the curled-up form in the bed a nearly inaudible reply came. "Yes, that's okay."

He firmly squeezed her left and right forearms and palpated her ankles and wrists. "Do you hurt here?"

"No, that's fine." When he pressed on the upper thighs, however, she cried out in pain. When he attempted to move the hips or shoulders she cried out, "Stop. Please STOP!"

We filed out of the room and gathered in a semicircle around Dr. Slocum. His gaze settled on me. "I think we can all agree that this poor woman is not hurting everywhere. I'm no rheumatologist, but I believe our patient has *polymyalgia rheumatica*, a painful immune system disorder of the hips and shoulders. I would hypothesize that her pain was so severe she became bedbound a few days prior to admission. Without adequate liquids she became dehydrated, and that led to her confusion. Not infection. Call lab and have them draw a sed rate and a C-reactive protein [laboratory tests which measure inflammation]. If they're markedly elevated, and I'm confident they will be, write an order for 15 mg of prednisone tonight and then daily. We'll start rounds here in the morning."

True to Slocum's prediction our patient's inflammation levels were sky high, and that evening she received her first dose of prednisone. Before leaving the hospital that night, I reviewed a medical journal article on *polymyalgia rheumatica* and committed to memory the clinical criteria: Age greater than 55, incapacitating pain and stiffness in both shoulders and hips, elevated inflammatory markers. Causation: unknown.

The next morning, sunlight beamed through an open window as I stopped by our patient's room a few minutes before Dr. Slocum was due to arrive. Remarkably, she was sitting up in a chair sipping a cup of tea and reading a book. The breakfast tray was empty. Her long gray hair was freshly washed and braided, and looking up, she gave me a sly grin. "I heard your group discussing my case out in the hallway yesterday and hoped that Dr. Slocum was correct. Oh my! Here he comes now!"

I stepped to the side as Dr. Slocum and the medical students silently filed into the room. Our poet patient slowly stood and gracefully touched her toes. Then she balanced first on one foot and then the other. I wondered if she was going to grab Dr. Slocum's hand and take him for a spin around the bed.

At the end of my internal medicine training, I knew that a rheumatology fellowship was not in the cards. I had been awarded a National Health Service Corps Scholarship in medical school, with the caveat that I practice in a physician shortage area. That's how I came to practice in Maine. Between 1985 and 1991, I traveled by boat and staffed clinics on Peaks and Chebeague Island with frequent house calls on Long Island and Cliff Island.

It was during this time of island-hopping and hospital rounds from my home on Peaks Island that my absent-mindedness re-emerged full-blown. Wallets were lost, coats and gloves abandoned on benches, car keys and boat keys woefully misplaced. In hopes of stemming the tide of lost items and missed appointments, I developed the habit of writing down reminders in my shirt pocket At-A-Glance weekly planner. Over time, I found myself jotting down reminders about reminders, a rabbit hole of forgetfulness. Sometimes it worked.

My pocket planner also captured interesting snippets of conversations and random ruminations. Here is a concise note from a surgeon on a woman whose left lower leg he had amputated following a diagnosis of cancer. *Acquired absence of left leg below knee.* Or these observations: *The more questions a patient has regarding side effects, the less likely they'll tolerate a prescribed medication.* And this: *The more supplements a patient takes, the more likely they will discontinue a prescription medication due to side effects.*

With only rudimentary laboratory testing at the Peaks Island and Chebeague Island clinics, arriving at a correct diagnosis was a constant challenge. Without an X-ray, how was I to decide if a patient's shortness of breath was from pneumonia or asthma? The chest pain from rib discomfort or heart disease? The weight loss due to depression or from an underlying cancer? I took to heart the lessons learned from my hospitalized elderly poet with *polymyalgia rheumatic* and relied on a careful, unhurried history and physical exam. When in doubt, and there were many occasions when I was in doubt, I drew blood for laboratory testing in Portland, or insisted that the patient take the ferry to the mainland for additional X-ray studies or consultation with a specialist.

That is, if the patient was willing to travel to the mainland. This was not always a given in this gritty, underserved population. When a patient did not take my advice, I was faced with three choices: refuse to take care of the patient; apply gentle pressure through family and friends until the patient agreed to additional tests; do the best I could with the tools I possessed. Eventually, most patients in need of further diagnostic testing or consultation with a specialist relented and took the ferry to town. Some did not.

This refinement in my "soft" persuasive skills held me in good stead when I became a rheumatologist.

Why did I eventually transition to rheumatology from primary care? Several years after we moved to Peaks Island, our second child, Molly, was born. Despite my vow to avoid the same fate as my father, I was working 70-80 hours each week, exercising less and less, and having difficulty sleeping through the night. Sandi and I went to marriage counseling. Nearly all of our recurring issues revolved around my long hours. Thankfully, I avoided my father's cigarette habit.

Then I had a real wake-up call. While trail running through the interior of Peaks Island, I developed vague chest pressure and became short of breath. Concerned, I stopped and stood still for a moment, unsure if what I had experienced was real. When I broke into a brisk run, the chest discomfort recurred. I felt for my pulse and it was racing. My breathing took several minutes before returning to baseline. I walked slowly home along the winding woodland path, acutely aware of my own fragile mortality.

The next day (if I'd had any sense, I would have gone to the emergency room—doctors make notoriously poor patients), I went to my doctor on the mainland, and in quick succession underwent an echocardiogram of my heart—abnormal, a treadmill –abnormal, and the following week, at age 35, a heart catheterization.

Somewhat surprisingly, the arteries supplying blood to my heart were completely normal, but my heart muscle had been weakened by a virus. This explained my symptoms. It could get better, the cardiologist shrugged, stay the same, or slowly decline. There were no medications to treat the condition, unless it worsened, and no way of predicting if I would recover. Assured that I was not in immediate danger of dying, I continued to slowly jog. Thankfully, over several years, my heart function gradually recovered and I was able to transition from jogging back to running.

My interest in autoimmune disorders continued to grow. Rheumatology cases on the islands seemed to percolate quietly in my mind, only to push into my consciousness at odd times: in the shower, on a midday lunch run, or on the ferry. Despite the demands of my island practice, I attended weekly Rheumatology Grand Rounds at Maine Medical Center in Portland, where I was able to share my most challenging cases. Following one particularly complex presentation, Dr. Paulding Phelps (a former president of the American College of Rheumatology) sat me down and suggested that I apply for a fellowship in rheumatology and offered to write a letter of recommendation. A year later, he repeated the offer. As an extra enticement, and convinced of the absolute necessity for my Finnish wife, Sandi, to enjoy a regular sauna, he gifted me his electric sauna. This clinched the deal.

Four months later, I was accepted in the Rheumatology and Clinical Immunology program at the University of Pittsburgh. My six years serving the Casco Bay Islands as a primary care doctor came to an end. Once again, Professor Andy Balber's basic immunology class at Bates College was directing my career path.

Chapter 4

"No drug is totally useless until it has been tried in scleroderma."

Attributed to Gerald Rodnan, MD

It was my first Tuesday as a rheumatology fellow at the University of Pittsburgh's Presbyterian University Hospital. Navigating a maze of buildings and hallways, I paused at the entrance to the scleroderma clinic and clicked open the door. All business in my white lab coat and lobster necktie, I focused on the gray carpet, aiming for a door adjacent to the check-in counter.

A cough caught my attention, and half-turning, I made eye contact with a middle-aged, emaciated woman whose woody face shook me to the bone. A loose afghan sweater draped over her boney shoulders. An intravenous line tunneled through her neck, delivering a creamy solution from a plastic bag hooked onto a stainless-steel pole. She smiled, but her mouth opened awkwardly, doll-like. Her smile was all teeth, the hidebound skin of her cheeks resisting the upward pull of her lips. I waved awkwardly back. She pulled a clawlike hand out from beneath the afghan and flexed the fingers in reply.

Inside, I shook hands with my preceptor, Thomas A. Medsger Jr., MD, a slender academic with thinning, gray hair and chief of the Department of Clinical Immunology and Rheumatology. He pushed his glasses back from where they rested at the tip of his nose, extended a hand, and glanced at his watch. "Good morning. Next time, please be here 15 minutes early. We have a busy day ahead. As a center for scleroderma patient care and research, these evaluations take a considerable amount of time.

"Remember, not every patient we consult on has scleroderma. There are scleroderma mimics. Myxomatous granulomatosis, and of course the eosinophilic myalgia syndrome, to name a few." I hoped my face didn't betray the fact that in my previous six years as a primary care internist, I'd never seen a case of scleroderma, much less—to my knowledge—a scleroderma mimic. "Be thorough," he added. "This is a multi-system disease. The skin changes can be heartbreaking, but the deeper involvement of the lungs, heart, bowels, and kidneys are where the most life-threatening damage may occur."

I pulled my first patient's chart from the rack: 42 years old, female, married, two children, from—I flipped back to the information page—Albuquerque, New Mexico. Geophysicist. That's interesting. There was a letter from her internist, a recent consult from the University of Arizona Arthritis Center, and reams of radiology and laboratory studies. I scribbled down notes for my presentation to Dr. Medsger. Then I knocked lightly on the door and entered. The woman I had waved to was my first patient, Dr. Jennifer Indura. She smiled again and introduced her husband, Michael. Up close, her appearance was even more disquieting; her face waxy and taut; the skin covering her forearms thickened and woody.

Together, we reviewed her recent history. "Last winter I went out to scrape ice off the windshield and forgot my mittens," she began. "The fingers turned white. They looked dead, like all the blood was drained out. My internist told me it was Raynaud's and started me on a medication. A few months later, even putting my hand into the freezer to take out a package of vegetables triggered an attack. That's when I began to get these."

Her husband gently removed a beige blanket from her lap, exposing her hands. The tip of the ring finger of the right hand was blackened and cold. The opposite hand was wrapped in a sterile dressing. She flinched as I gently tried to unwrap the gauze. Reflexively, her husband leaned forward and put his hand over mine. "Here, let me help you." He reached into his wife's handbag and pulled out a pint of sterile water to soak the gauze, then applied a dab of anesthetic cream to the base of the finger. "That should make it easier to remove. Let's wait a few minutes."

There was an awkward silence. Now I've done it. Five minutes into my first consult as a rheumatology fellow and I've already broken the Hippocratic Oath: *Do no harm.* I looked up from my notes and steadied my voice. "After the Raynaud's, then what happened?"

"It was strange, but several weeks later the fingers became puffy and swollen and my hands nearly unusable. That's when I took a leave of absence from my teaching position at the University of Arizona. I was referred to a rheumatologist who told me it looked like I had early scleroderma." She reached up and scratched her forehead with her free hand, winced and shifted slightly. "She changed out the Raynaud's medications and that helped a little, but at our follow-up visit, they told me there wasn't any treatment that can prevent the skin tightening."

Our eyes met and I allowed myself, for a moment, to imagine what it must be like to find myself encased in skin so thickened and tight it restricted simple movement. I consciously slowed my breathing. If I was to help manage her illness, I needed to maintain some distance. Empathy is critically important but not if it overwhelms objectivity. I maintained eye contact but shifted my focus to the details of how her disease had progressed.

"I think you can take that last roll of gauze off now," she nodded. "I'm okay."

As I reached over and unwrapped the dressing, she jerked her hand away and cried out. A sliver of scab and a chunk of deeper gray tissue came off with the gauze. The blackened finger looked raw and painful but no blood seeped from the wound. My first impression was that the tip of the finger should be amputated. It looked that bad. "Sorry," I said, loosely rewrapping the wound, "let's protect the finger." My throat was dry. I sucked on the inside of my cheeks, intensely aware of my patient's discomfort.

Her husband lightly held her hand and applied another dab of anesthetic to the wound. Dr. Indura closed her eyes for a moment before continuing. "The skin thickened and tightened. First the fingers and toes, then the back of my hands, forearms and ankles, more recently, the neck and face. I got depressed. I mean, I am depressed, can't sleep."

"Cough? Shortness of breath?" I asked

"No, but I really can't do much. Well, that's not really accurate. If I walk up a flight of stairs, I have to stop halfway up and catch my breath."

"And the weight loss? It looks like from your internist's notes, that you've lost about 30 pounds in the past six months?"

"That's stabilized," her husband interjected, looking through his notes. "She's the same weight as when they admitted her several months ago at the University of Arizona. The scleroderma has affected the bowel. She's not absorbing solid food normally."

"When a feeding tube didn't work out, that's when they placed this." Dr. Indura pointed to the right side of her neck where an IV tunneled beneath the skin, "The cream-colored fluids are fats. Lately, with some of the other medications they prescribed, I've been able to join the family for meals. Last week I enjoyed a few mouthfuls of my daughter's birthday cake, but if I eat more, I get this ungodly cramping and bloating." She exhaled and looked down at her hand. "It's been extraordinarily difficult."

Her husband touched her at her elbow. "Jennifer, do you think it's time for a Vicodin?" She silently nodded. He opened a bottle of water and placed two pills in her mouth.

Momentarily, I looked away. Dr. Indura was no longer an intellectual rising star in geophysics, but a patient with a progressive illness as disfiguring as leprosy. The scleroderma was like a slow-moving cancer, spreading from one vital organ to the next. I recalled a fragment of a poem on scleroderma that I had come across the night before as I had prepped for my first day of clinic.

> "It held me in its toxic vice,
> Slowly crushing dazzling life.
> From every cell it prodded and poked,
> Burnt and choked, the very soul of me…"
>
> Sam M. Morgan

Moving on, searching for anything that might distract me from the pathos of the visit, I ran my finger down the intake sheet. "Your blood pressure. 138/88. It's slightly elevated. Is that new?"

Her husband scratched the stubble on his cheek and flipped through his notes, seemingly relieved to be returning to a world of numbers. "Let me see, we don't check it very often at home. Two months ago, 112/74, three weeks ago, 140/86."

"Thanks." I reached over and felt Dr. Indura's forearms. I'd never felt scleroderma skin before. The sensation was disquieting, alien, reptilian. The thickened tissue resisted my attempts to gather a fleshy portion between my thumb and forefinger. Both hands had a disquieting clawlike appearance.

Dr. Indura cocked her head and asked, "Have you been in your rheumatology training program very long?" There was a pause, a dropped beat in our conversation. No longer a patient, she was once again a Professor of Geophysics, probing, following her instincts, asking hard questions.

"As a matter of fact," I exhaled slowly, "this is my first day." The jig was up, the imposter unmasked. Paradoxically, I felt more at ease. She was the professor. I was the student. I felt my neck muscles loosen.

Dr. Indura pointed to my white mustache, "You look a little old for a student. I thought for a moment that you were Dr. Medsger."

"I practiced internal medicine for a number of years in Maine before applying to the fellowship program here at Pitt, but there's no question, I'm starting over again."

"Well, as you can see, I'm not your usual introductory case," she raised an eyebrow. "More like the final exam." Our relationship reset, I continued my exam. When I was finished, I walked back to the doctors' station, sat down across from Dr. Medsger, and summarized Dr. Indura's story beginning with the Raynaud's, the fingertip ulcers, the progressive hidebound skin, the weight loss, the placement of the intravenous line for nutrition. I was about to …

"Blood pressure?" Dr. Medsger interjected. "We begin with the vital signs here." He paused. "They're important."

I looked down at my notes. "Blood pressure 138/88, pulse 82 per minute. But she's anxious and in pain. Her husband has recorded several normal blood pressures, so today's reading might be a red herring, a blip."

"Or?" Dr. Medsger asked quietly.

I blinked. Suddenly, it came to me. "Scleroderma hypertension."

"Could be." Dr. Medsger replied. "Did you repeat it?"

"No, but her blood pressure is only borderline elevated, isn't it? In my former internal medicine practice, I wouldn't even consider medications unless the readings were consistently over 140/90."

Without a word, Dr. Medsger reached into his briefcase and pulled out a recent article from the *Journal of Medicine* and plunked it on the table. Dr. Medsger was the lead author. He cleared his throat and pointed to the summary. "You'll find several patients in this review with blood pressures in Dr. Indura's range. What's more, scleroderma hypertension is often resistant to many commonly used blood pressure medications. Only aggressive management with medications from the ACE inhibitor family can prevent these patients from going on to kidney failure and requiring dialysis."

I wondered if he was going to ask me to go back to Maine.

Dr. Medsger handed me the article, stood, and buttoned his white coat. "Anything else?"

"Her lungs. Crackles are present halfway up both lung fields." I hesitated before asking, "Could she have scleroderma lung disease?"

"This would be the right setting. Good. Very good. Let's take a look."

Entering the room, Dr. Medsger gently patted Dr. Indura's forearm and asked if he could see a picture of her two children. A crooked smile radiated across her face. With painstaking effort, she opened up her purse with the better of her two hands and retrieved a photo of the girls on ice skates flanking their father.

"Beautiful girls. Ice skating in Albuquerque—who would guess?" Dr. Medsger handed back the picture and repeated Dr. Indura's blood pressure. "We'll take it again in a few minutes. Dr. Radis, can you ask Gail at the front desk to call the laboratory?"

A few minutes later, the phlebotomist knocked on our door, and drew six tubes of blood. In a low voice, Dr. Medsger pointed to a red top tube and requested that the samples be run STAT. For the next fifteen minutes, he assessed where and to what degree scleroderma had thickened and transformed the skin. Following this, he focused his attention on the lungs, where I had reported significant abnormalities.

Concluding his exam, he drew a graph with a single curved line. The line rose steeply, leveled out and ever so slowly declined. "This," Dr. Medsger declared to the Induras, "is what we believe is the natural history of diffuse scleroderma. In the first one to two years, skin thickness increases rapidly. After that, skin thickening slows or even improves somewhat."

I was only too aware of what he omitted, that while the disease may stop progressing, the internal damage is usually permanent, and that nearly 40% of patients die during the first seven years. He met Dr. Indura's eyes and continued. "What they undoubtedly told you at the University of Arizona is that there is no medical treatment that has been shown to slow down or reverse scleroderma, and unfortunately, that's true. But we have a number of experimental trials here at the University of Pittsburgh looking at promising medications in early scleroderma."

"Am I still early?" Dr. Indura asked.

"Yes. Despite your rapidly progressive disease, you would be a candidate for one of our studies." There was a knock on the door and Dr. Medsger was handed Dr. Indura's laboratory results.

"Is there a problem?" Dr. Indura asked.

"We'd like you to stay here at the hospital for a few days," Dr. Medsger replied evenly. "Your elevated blood pressure is having an effect on the function of your kidneys. We need to aggressively..."

At this, Dr. Indura burst into tears. She'd managed the flight from Arizona, the cramped seating and awkward transfers from the plane to a rental car to the hotel, a leaking connector to her intravenous line, and the news that the University of Pittsburgh didn't have a magic bullet for her scleroderma. Now, she was being told that her kidneys were damaged. She lay her head on her husband's shoulder and sobbed.

According to a paper published in the Annals of Internal Medicine by Gerald P. Rodnan, MD, and Thomas G. Benedek, MD, the first convincing account of scleroderma can be found in a monograph described by Carlo Curzio in 1753. "*...a young woman, seventeen years old...with a complaint of excessive tension and hardness of the skin over all her body, by which she found herself so bound and straiten'd, that she could barely move her limbs...her skin hard to the touch, like wood, or a dry hide.*"

Treatment consisted of warm milk, vapor baths, blood-letting, and small doses of oral mercury. Miraculously, over the course of eleven months, the young woman made a complete recovery. Since modern-day treatment of scleroderma almost never results in a cure, either the description was of a scleroderma mimic and resolved spontaneously, or the mercury somehow disrupted the abnormal underpinnings of the disease without fatally poisoning the patient.

Causation of scleroderma has been equally perplexing. On the one hand, certain occupations with chronic exposure to chemicals such as polyvinyl chloride or benzene raises the risk in men for developing the disease. But this fails to explain why only a tiny fraction of men in these occupations develop scleroderma. What's more, any hypothesis regarding environmental triggers must account for the fact that the vast majority of cases of diffuse scleroderma are in women with no obvious toxic chemical exposure. Additional insights into the trigger(s) for diffuse scleroderma have been difficult to tease out. Genetic predisposition may play a role, but with an estimated annual incidence of only 19 cases per million, other factors beyond genetic risk undoubtably play a role.

After clinic hours, I located Dr. Indura in the intensive care unit. She was asleep, nestled in a matrix of intravenous lines. A plastic tube was taped to her nose and provided her with supplemental oxygen. A vase held several roses. On her bed table was the picture of her husband and two daughters on ice skates.

Her nurse met me outside the room. "She's had a difficult morning. Her blood pressure is running high. The medical student, resident and medicine attending took a long time to settle her in, and she just dozed off. And you are?" She glanced down at my name tag.

"Chuck Radis. I'm the new rheumatology fellow."

“We don’t see you guys down here very often.” She glanced back at the curtain. “Her skin looks awful. Have you seen her fingers? They look like they’re going to fall off.”

I decided not to answer her question directly. “So did the primary service read my clinic note and start her on captopril for the hypertension?”

“Let me see.” She scanned the med list. “Okay, here it is, 25 mg of captopril twice daily. I gave her the first dose about 30 minutes ago. Poor thing, she’s so young to have kidney failure. The medicine service is worried the captopril might bottom out her blood pressure and worsen her kidney function, so they’re taking it slow.”

Having quickly reviewed Dr. Medsger’s article on scleroderma hypertension, I knew this was absolutely the wrong approach. “Can you get me the beeper number of the resident? From our perspective, we need to push the dose up quickly to normalize her blood pressure, otherwise her kidneys are going to completely shut down. Has her blood pressure been running this high all day?” I asked.

“No, but creeping pretty steadily upward. So have her oxygen needs. What’s going on there?”

“We think the scleroderma has affected her lungs.”

At that moment, Dr. Medsger strode through the door and peeked through the curtain at Dr. Indura. Glancing at the blood pressure monitor, he turned on his heels and addressed me in a clipped tone. “Dr. Radis, what’s going on with her blood pressure medications?”

“First dose 30 minutes ago.”

“That’s unacceptable. Have you called the primary service?” The ICU nurse quietly dialed the internal medicine resident’s pager. A moment later I was on the phone with the resident and making the case, no, telling the resident Dr. Indura needed more aggressive blood pressure management. Now.

When I looked up, Dr. Medsger was sitting on the edge of Dr. Indura's bed. The pharmacy drawer at the nursing station was open. He wasn't about to wait. "Dr. Indura, I want you to take an additional dose of this blood pressure medication." The pill dropped off her fingertips onto the floor. Unwrapping another pill, he placed it onto her palm. "Take your time. Dr. Radis, can you get us a cup of water? Let's make sure it goes all the way down." He remained silent as she swallowed the pill and wearily settled back in bed.

He pulled up a chair and opened her medical chart. "The pill we've started is critically important in controlling your high blood pressure, and we'll be titrating up the dose until your blood pressure normalizes. Over time, we expect your kidneys will slowly improve. But that may take many months." He paused and pulled out her chest X-ray from a folder and hung it on the view box on the far wall. "And I'm sorry, but there's more bad news. These patchy white areas are likely triggered by your scleroderma. It's why you now require supplemental oxygen. I've consulted one of our pulmonary specialists. I'm recommending they perform a bronchoscopy, a test where they pass a flexible tube into your windpipe to biopsy the lung."

During the night, Dr. Indura's blood pressure continued to climb, at one point reaching 210/118. When we reached the maximum recommended dose of the first medication, a second medication was added, and still the pressures remained uncontrolled. Over the next day, the pointer and ring finger of the right hand blackened and turned stone cold. A morphine drip was hung and she was able to sleep through the next night. Her kidney function continued to deteriorate.

Surgery declared that the pointer finger would need to be amputated at the middle knuckle, but the patient was too unstable to operate. Dermatology performed a forearm skin biopsy for a research study. A lung specialist passed a bronchoscope into the lungs to clarify whether an unusual infection was affecting the lungs or active scleroderma. Following the lung procedure, Dr. Indura's oxygen levels never returned to baseline. She became increasingly short of breath and restless, requiring a mild tranquilizer.

That night Dr. Indura's lungs filled with fluid and her oxygen levels plummeted. When I made my early morning rounds, I heard the rhythmic whoosh of the ventilator before I pulled open the curtain to her room. I went out to talk with her husband. He was alone in the family room, his eyes puffy and bloodshot. I sat down and lightly patted him on the shoulder.

"Medsger? Is he around yet this morning?"

"No. Not yet. It's 6:00 a.m. He usually rounds by 7:00," I replied.

I offered Mr. Indura a Snicker's bar. We ate together in silence. "Why Jennifer?" he glanced towards her room. "I've been reading what I can in the medical library, but I don't get it. Our backyard backs up onto a national forest. We don't use chemicals on our lawn. She eats right, doesn't smoke or do drugs. No one else in her extended family has an autoimmune disease. She's brilliant, speaks at research conferences around the world, works like a dog, great mother," his voice cracked. "Great wife."

"I know, it doesn't make sense," I agreed.

"She's like Job. Every inch of her body seems like it's encased by scleroderma. And inside, now her bowel, the lung, the kidneys are shutting down." His hand was shaking as he finished the Snicker's bar. "Is this some sort of cosmic payback?"

The following day, I attended our weekly 7 a.m. rheumatology conference. The room was overflowing with basic science researchers, rheumatologists, pulmonary specialists, and rheumatology fellows. A pathologist reviewed the lung biopsy slides of Dr' Indura on an overhead screen. Over the green expanse of three blackboards, arrows and lines connected the possible regulatory pathways of the immune system leading to scleroderma. Communication pathways between cells were presented as a rogue's gallery of potential triggers of the disease that could be targeted for novel drug studies.

I copied the blackboard presentation in my pocket calendar to review at home.

The senior fellow on our consulting team caught my attention and handed me a folded piece of paper. Opening the note, it read: *Dr. Indura has passed away. Autopsy at four today. New scleroderma consult room 631. Talk to me after conference.*

I slumped into the chair and ran my fingers through my hair. I knew that Dr. Indura had been critically ill, but passed away? I looked over to Dr. Medsger. He picked up a piece of chalk and circled a particularly promising pathway in the treatment of scleroderma on the blackboard. As one of the world's leading experts on scleroderma, what must it be like to have so many patients die under your care? Our eyes met for a moment. He knew. Tapping the board for emphasis, he said, "Any more questions? If not, let's get back to work."

That night, I dreamed I was in a glider silently cruising over a city, low enough to make out clusters of pedestrians crowding the sidewalks. Everywhere I looked amid the bustle of the city there was chaos, but amid the chaos there was a sense of purpose and order. Trucks spewed exhaust fumes, taxis beeped. A fire truck roared by to put out a fire. The light changed. A surge of humanity crossed the street. Construction crews stood by open manhole covers ready to descend into a maze of pipes and electrical conduits. Beneath the streets, hidden from view, fluids coursed through water and septic lines, nourishing and flushing the system of toxic wastes.

Like a city, the body's immune system is held together by complex checks and balances. Under the guidance of specialized cells, the system up-regulates and down-regulates with astounding precision to fight infection or eliminate early cells of malignancy. Then something goes wrong, and the immune system attacks the thyroid (as in Hashimoto's thyroiditis), the insulin-secreting cells of the pancreas (as in Type 1 diabetes), or, in the case of scleroderma, the skin, lungs, bowel, and heart.

Dr. Medsger at the University of Pittsburgh and others around the globe have devoted entire medical careers to chasing down leads, performing clinical trials, incrementally improving the care for this dreadful disease. For now, the mystery of scleroderma remains. I remember Dr. Indura.

Chapter 5

Rheumatologist:
A physician with specialized training in inflammatory disease.

Rheumatologist:
(Overheard in the doctor's dining room).
A clinician who comes to the bedside, orders a lot of tests which come back inconclusive
and treats the patient with steroids.

Following the completion of my rheumatology fellowship in Pittsburgh, our family returned to our home on Peaks Island in the summer of 1993. As much as I enjoyed the friendships I made at Pitt, to become a member of the faculty would have required an additional degree in Public Health or a basic science PhD in immunology. At heart I was not an academic with its mix of patient care, research, administrative responsibilities, and frequent faculty meetings. My niche in medicine was in full-time patient care and rheumatologists were in short supply in Maine, numbering only twelve in the entire state. It was a decision I've never regretted.

Arriving in Maine after a long day's drive from Pittsburgh, we drove our rental van onto the car ferry in Portland and off-loaded onto Peaks Island 25 minutes later. I parked the van across the street from the candy store, and before indulging in an ice cream cone, third-grader Kate and first-grader Molly crouched down unexpectantly and kissed the ground. Sandi was beaming. The poignancy of the moment was plain.

I became the fifth rheumatologist at Rheumatology Associates, about a twenty-minute drive from where the ferry docked in Portland. Living and commuting from an unbridged year-round island in Maine can be challenging. While hourly ferries conveniently leave Peaks early each morning, the problems mount on the return trip. Peaks Islanders with jobs on the mainland board either the 5:35, 7:15, or 8:15 evening ferry. This meant that if you narrowly missed the 5:35 ferry, instead of arriving home at six p.m., it was closer to eight.

Ri Ra's, an Irish bar adjacent to the ferry terminal, was a favorite watering hole for frustrated commuters missing the 5:35 ferry home. Guinness beer was on tap and Irish staples such as shepherd's pie and bangers and mash were on the menu. I like beer, but to improve the likelihood that I arrived home before bedtime to play with our young children, I planned to commute year-round—weather permitting—in my 16-foot boat, SAKAMO (SAndi, KAte, MOlly) rather than by ferry. This meant motoring across the bay during the winter months when ice flows dot the harbor. Of course, living in Maine also means coming and going in the dark for four months of the year and dealing with snow and high winds.

Having previously owned a boat, I believed that I could commute from Peaks in relative safety. A former merchant marine patient of mine, Bud Peary, summed up the learning curve for boating in Maine succinctly: *You haven't learned anything until you've sunkyour first boat.* Luckily, I'd already sunk my first boat (I was not on it at the time) and I felt confident I could put those lessons to good use. Convincing my wife, Sandi, that I could safely commute back and forth to Portland was another matter. Ultimately, she was able to separate the hapless absent-minded husband she knew all too wel, from the focused, responsible waterman I could someday be. Even I, perhaps, was capable of following a strict routine.

To commute to Portland in SAKAMO, the following check-list was required: Drive my truck to the pier and leave the keys next to the stick shift for Sandi. Climb down a 14-foot iron ladder to my float, safely board and don my life preserver. Next, switch on the battery, then my running lights and check the fuel tanks before lowering the engine into the water. Flip on the marine radio, start the engine. Only then would I clamber out of the boat to release the lines, reboard, and point SAKAMO towards Portland.

In winter, releasing the lines from the cleats was complicated by waves washing onto my float and forming ice deposits on the lines. This required using a hammer to break up the ice on the cleat. From time to time, ice and snow accumulated inside the boat and this meant using my hammer to shatter the ice on the deck of SAKAMO, a disconcerting image to a casual observer. These last two maneuvers Sandi was not fully aware of.

At Rheumatology Associates, I bonded with George Morton, MD, who, if this were possible, seemed to be even more disorganized than me. His charts were stacked 10 deep on his desk and on the floor, and laboratory and X-ray reports were strewn haphazardly on chairs or along the back shelf. I say seemed to be more disorganized because unlike my daily struggle to locate most everything, Dr. Morton never seemed to misplace a thing; he knew where every chart and every piece of paper in his office resided. I envied his disorganized competence.

Rheumatologists are specialists in arthritis and systemic immunologic disorders and not every patient with joint pain belongs in our office. Picture an arthritis patient and you most likely visualize your grandmother's bony fingers, or an elderly man shuffling along with a cane. But this type of arthritis, osteoarthritis, doesn't require a consultation with a rheumatologist. In most cases, I have nothing to offer these patients beyond what their own primary care practitioner can offer: medications for pain, an occasional cortisone injection, an orthopedic referral for joint replacement.

It is the mysterious world of more than 100 immunologic and rare metabolic and genetic disorders which rheumatologists are, at their core, trained to recognize and treat. Our tools are medications which suppress or modulate the immune system; our goal, to reduce or eliminate pain, maintain function, and prevent damage. We are the doctors of rare diseases, illnesses which may affect 1 in 10,000 or 1 in 100,000 patients, or are known only by a handful of case reports in the literature. Eponyms for these diseases fill our daily discourse: Behcet's disease, Sjogren's syndrome, Still's disease, Takayasu's arteritis, Kikuchi's syndrome, Moyamoya disease.

Every physician brings their own idiosyncrasies to the practice of medicine. Some of my quirks date back to my years in primary care. From my desk behind the front counter at the Peaks Island Health Center (a winterized cottage donated to the community), I could see everyone in the waiting room. When my nurse led my next patient to an exam room, I quietly noted their balance and gait. Were they limping? In pain? Did they appear anxious or depressed?

As a rheumatologist, I continued this habit and added several others. Before I see my next patient, I review the medication list. Why? Some medication side effects may mimic autoimmune disease. Statins, drugs commonly prescribed to reduce cholesterol, may cause muscle aching and weakness. Several cardiology medications may trigger drug-induced lupus. Even supplements need to be carefully scrutinized; at times, their ingestion may be associated with joint inflammation. Thankfully, these side effects gradually resolve with discontinuation of the offending drug.

It is addition by subtraction; a return to health by removing the triggering drug.

Following this—again, before I enter the room—I review my new consult's list of comorbidities (medical parlance for the presence of two or more diseases). If the patient is taking a half-dozen medications for, say, diabetes, sleep apnea, congestive heart failure, and depression, my job is to assess whether a new disease is hiding in plain sight. Symptoms of autoimmune disease such as fatigue, muscle aching, and joint pain, are shared by a multitude of conditions, including two of the conditions listed above: sleep apnea and depression.

Lastly, I evaluate the results of previous laboratory testing. In rheumatology, some of our most commonly ordered laboratory tests, the anti-nuclear antibody (ANA) and rheumatoid factor (RF), are seen not only in those with autoimmune disorders, but in viral illnesses, and in healthy patients with an aging immune system. How common is a false positive ANA? By age 65, as many as 10% of the population may have a detectable ANA on laboratory analysis. Don't get me going on the lack of significance of a low-level positive rheumatoid factor.

Rheumatology practice is still decidedly low-tech. A comprehensive history and physical exam are as important to us today as it was for physicians 50 years ago. With rare exceptions, we have no "gold standard" test which is 100% predictive of a specific disease. Instead, we live in a world of lab results which must be interpreted alongside the evidence we've gathered in our history and physical. In rheumatology, making a difficult diagnosis is similar to a trial in which evidence is presented to a jury. The rheumatologist is tasked with assessing the strength of the evidence. A guilty verdict (the diagnosis) is a judgment that there is no alternative explanation for the evidence.

The "art" of medicine is alive and well in rheumatology.

In recent years, even as the electronic medical record (EMR) has supplanted paper charts, I generally refuse to use it while in the exam room. My recording tools are a clipboard and a printout of the afternoon's schedule on which I jot down notes. Adjacent to each patient's name on the printout is a miniature skeleton homunculus where I can darken in particular joints that are painful or swollen.

I often draw arrows and question marks connecting symptoms and physical findings. Some of my notations are random quotes that help me recall other details of the case. "*At age 80, loves to roller skate!*" or "*under chronic stress from son's drug addiction,*" or "*beloved dog, Mitch, died,*" critical but often overlooked insights into a patient's psychological health.

It's important for me to make eye contact, particularly when I am trying to convince a patient to take a medication with potentially dangerous side effects. Typing while looking at a screen makes this impossible. Eye contact tells my patient that I'm truly interested in their story. It builds trust, and perhaps improves the likelihood that they will follow my advice. Only when I return to my office do I summarize the visit in the EMR.

Whenever possible, I keep my notes brief and to the point. Among medical providers, it's well known that the EMR has become a billing tool full of nonessential fluff to justify a higher billing code for payment from health insurance companies. These office visit notes may stretch over ten or eleven pages for a simple examination. Because most of my career has been in private practice, I can refuse to participate in this expensive, time-consuming shell game. In this way, the time I spend with my patients is a respite in my day rather than a soul-draining troika between the computer, myself, and the unfortunate patient.

On a typical rheumatology day in the office, I usually see 15 follow-up patients and two to four consults. Thankfully, many of my follow-up visits are routine. The diagnosis is firmly established and the patient has adjusted to living with a chronic illness. The medications are working well. The ulcerating rash has healed; the inflammation in the lungs, joints, brain, or heart has resolved. Cautious optimism has replaced painful uncertainty. Fatigue, an elusive symptom that is pervasive in rheumatologic practice, is better.

We chat amicably during these routine visits as I address the patient's concerns and review recent laboratory results. I explain the Goldilocks approach to medications in rheumatology: This dose is too high. This dose too low. This dose is just right. Patients often tease me that my tie looks like I chose it in the dark. We laugh.

Not every follow-up patient in my practice is doing well. There are some patients I see who don't respond to standard immunologic treatments. Or, alternatively, if a patient improves, side effects may force me to discontinue a beneficial medication and substitute a less effective drug. In these cases, ongoing pain may be the cause of frequent absences from work. There may be applications for me to fill out for handicap parking or Social Security Disability Insurance, or questions regarding whether the patient qualifies for a low-cost medication program. If a spouse or friend attends, I shift my attention to answer their additional questions as best I can. I try to remain optimistic.

But like all physicians I have my moments. I do not always remain fully engaged and empathetic. No physician does 100% of the time. There are some patients I simply don't connect with. As the visit drags on, my stomach churns. My neck aches. Emotionally charged visits take time and if I am already running behind, I have to make a conscious effort to maintain my focus.

If after several visits, a diagnosis remains in doubt, I may discuss the case at Rheumatology Grand Rounds at Maine Medical Center. There, I share my most puzzling cases with other rheumatologists, medical residents, internists, a radiologist, and several orthopedic surgeons. One of my partners may recall a particularly vexing patient with similar symptoms and suggest that testing for A, B, or C may clarify the diagnosis. These weekly conferences are excellent learning experiences and play an important role in making all of us better diagnosticians.

From time to time, I refer patients to the Massachusetts General Hospital, in Boston, Presbyterian University Hospital in Pittsburgh, or the Cleveland Clinic. These rheumatology consultants see the rarest of the rare diseases, and reviewing their notes is like attending a master class. But even at these institutions, there are times when a specific diagnosis cannot be made.

Where do patients go for a third or fourth opinion? A handful of my patients have been evaluated at the Undiagnosed Disease Program at the National Institute of Health in Bethesda, Maryland where they may be admitted for an intensive workup. Multiple specialties collaborate to clarify an elusive diagnosis. But even here, a specific diagnosis is not always forthcoming. Despite recent advances in genetic sequencing looking for mutations associated with rare diseases, despite the experience of some of the country's top specialists, some patients simply do not fit into a specific diagnostic category.

Thankfully, this doesn't mean that the patient continues to suffer. A trial of an immunosuppressant medication may be recommended, oftentimes with dramatic improvement in their mystery illness. One of my longtime patients, whom I have followed without a firm diagnosis for the better part of a decade, refers to herself as a "mysterioma," but thankfully is in remission on immunotherapy.

When I initially don't know what is wrong with a sick patient, their story stays with me long after their office visit is over. I am, if anything, persistent. Thankfully, the weight of this connection doesn't usually carry over to my home life or interfere with sleep. Instead, difficult cases percolate in my subconscious, what researchers have described as the deliberation without attention effect. When my subconscious rehashes a puzzling case, it's not unusual for me to awaken in the morning—or occasionally in the middle of the night—with new insights. This phenomenon may also occur while I am running or hiking or out for an evening walk.

I have learned to acknowledge and appreciate these suggestions. They are, after all, coming from…me. If my pocket planner is handy, I write them down in tiny cursive before they retreat into my subconscious. And honestly, not all of these insights pan out. I am not a medical savant.

From time to time, I consult on patients with severe, sometimes untreated mental illness, who may also have rheumatic symptoms. This complicates the picture. Unexplained, life-altering pain is common in patients with mental illness. In some cases, the symptoms are related to anxiety or depression or post-traumatic stress disorder. In others, the pain may be due to an unexplained autoimmune disease or cancer. The challenge is to sift through the symptoms and determine a diagnosis. These are difficult, complex visits.

One busy afternoon, I noticed that Joanne had taped a note to the back of my office chair after she checked in a new patient. The note simply said: *Man in exam room #3 has a gun.* I reread the note. Maine has a rich hunting tradition and liberal open carry laws. If the man posed a threat, I am sure Joanne would have knocked on my door and interrupted me. Wouldn't she have?

Joanne was nowhere to be seen, so I knocked on the door and smiled pleasantly at a very large man (on the north side of 300 pounds) seated on the exam table wearing an undershirt and jeans. Through the undershirt I could make out a dark strap wrapped around his chest. On his flank was a distinctive bulge. I decided to address the issue head-on. "Good afternoon. Before we get started, I see that you're carrying a handgun. Here in Maine, there is no law prohibiting you from bringing a gun into our office," I paused to assess his reaction, "but I'd appreciate it if you'd go back outside and lock the gun in your vehicle."

"You mean this?" he reached beneath his T-shirt and pulled out a .357 Magnum and laid it on a small table between us. "I've got a permit. It's for my own protection. I'm a private investigator. Some pretty crazy stuff going on lately."

"Okay," I said uncertainly. My new patient did not appear to be in a hurry to part with his firearm. I was not of a mind to insist. "What can I do for you?"

"I'm here because I hurt all over," he continued, as I stared at the handgun. "My doctor referred me to you, hoping you can sort things out. Can't sleep. Bad headaches. Well, I probably sleep, but I'm driving my new girlfriend crazy with my snoring. She wakes up and shakes me because she claims I stop breathing. My doctor saw me last month and drew a lot of tests but all of them are normal. Yesterday I was so tired I blacked out driving. Some whacko almost rear-ended me. Sometimes I can't even think straight."

Then he leaned in and whispered, "I'm helping a lady friend up the road from where I live. She's in mortal danger. I have her stashed out on a mountaintop an hour from here. I keep hearing some guys are closing in on her. You know, the guys in the news. I think they're on to me. I have the area booby-trapped."

I stared back at him, considering this deluge of information. Sleep apnea was almost certainly present, but would need to be confirmed by a sleep study. Patients with sleep apnea often have widespread muscle aching, daytime drowsiness, and normal laboratory testing. I excused myself, backed out of the room, and called his family doctor. We both agreed that if Mr. A fell asleep at the wheel and got in an accident, having a loaded .357 Magnum on his hip was a recipe for disaster. Yes, his doctor would arrange for a sleep study. No, he didn't know the patient well, only met him twice.

When I returned to the room, the man was gone. Joanne called the police department in the town listed on his patient questionnaire. There was no record that a man by his name had applied for a concealed weapon permit. No, the police said, he wasn't on their list of private investigators. I never saw the man again, nor did his family doctor. He simply disappeared.

Five minutes later, I was on to my next scheduled patient. Is it any wonder that your doctor sometimes appears preoccupied?

This is why, no matter how far behind I am in clinic, whether my last visit went smoothly or was akin to having a tooth pulled without anesthetic, I take a moment between patients and clear my mind. Outside the doorway, I pull my next patient's record from the chart rack, scan their medication list and reacquaint myself with the details of their history. When I feel my jaw soften and my neck and shoulders unwind, I slowly exhale and open the door. Be sharp. It's time for another story.

Chapter 6

"You know, pigs are pigs. They eat most anything, and as long as you shovel their shit and keep their shed clean, they're pretty content."
Leon Withers.

In most of my unknown cases, it's not that I'm completely adrift. I've ruled out a host of conditions. I know that there doesn't appear to be cancer in the background or infection. I've excluded a number of genetic and autoimmune disorders. Even so, one of my most difficult tasks at a follow-up visit is to adjust my glasses, look the patient in the eye, and admit that I don't know what's wrong.

Such was the case with Leon Withers. At our first visit, I strolled past the partially open door to his exam room and peeked inside. He was unshaven, his hair a greasy black tangle. A faded, plaid Mackinaw wool shirt hung loosely over his chest and flowed over faded blue jeans. His grimy steel-toed work-boots were half-laced. The smell of smoke from his woodstove drifted into the hallway.

According to his referral doctor's notes, Mr. Withers's current weight of 238 pounds was down 20 pounds. Low grade fevers and sweats, sometime severe enough to change his T-shirt, occurred nightly. His hands hurt. His back and left knee ached. Under chief complaint he had written, *feel like sh*t, think I'm dying.*

The pig farmer's medical history was a long and rocky road. He was a chronic hepatitis C virus carrier, presumably from a borrowed needle shooting up heroin in his 20s, or maybe from the blood transfusions he required after a motorcycle accident some years later. Chronic back pain and a damaged knee left him with a permanent limp. On his medical questionnaire, after checking off diabetes, high blood pressure, and kidney stones, he circled depression with the notation: *Wouldn't you be?*

His family doctor had ordered every possible test. Spray and pray, we call it. The problem is, nearly all the tests came back borderline abnormal. This had led to further testing and more borderline abnormal results. Nothing seemed to add up. Looking up at the clock, I brought myself back to the problem at hand. When all else fails, the saying goes, examine the patient.

The first thing I noticed when I shook Mr. Withers's hand was that at the corner of his elbow, folded neatly at the crease, was a completed New York Times crossword puzzle, in ink. Put that into the mix, I thought. He cautiously extended his hand. "Thanks for not gripping too hard Doc, my fingers are killing me. You can call me Leon." An internal medicine resident who was spending a month-long rotation in my office lingered outside the door. Some patients are reluctant to have another doctor sit in on their consultation, but Leon was comfortable with the attention. "Come on in," he motioned, "two heads are better than one."

With a look of relief, the resident entered and leaned against the sink. For the past week, this particular third-year resident, Dr. Litmus, had shown that she was a cut above most of the residents who rotated through my office. She was comfortable with patients, bright, logical, and keenly engaged in patient care, and I was hoping to interest her in applying for a fellowship in rheumatology rather than her stated interest in cardiology. While introductions were made, I realized that my wallet was missing from my back pocket. I wondered if my nurse Joanne might loan me money for lunch. With a growing sense of apprehension, I reached into my front right pocket for my boat keys. Nothing. Maybe I left the keys in the ignition on SAKAMO? Maybe. It was dark when I came across the bay this morning.

I asked Leon how long he'd lived in Maine. "Five years. When my old man died, I came back to live with my mom, help out with the farm. My opportunities for making a living in New Jersey were what I would call, limited," he shrugged. "Prison will do that."

"What's it like working with pigs?"

"Yeah… You know, pigs are pigs. They eat most anything, and as long as you shovel their shit and keep their shed clean, they're pretty content. Seasonally, I tar driveways. Money's actually pretty good. Keeps me out of trouble."

"So, what was the first thing you noticed when your health changed?"

"Fatigue. That was early last summer, maybe five months ago. The heat and I don't agree so when I began to get the sweats at night, I didn't think much of it at first. But I got so bone-tired it was all I could do to drag myself out of bed." He stopped for a moment and scratched at his elbow. "I think the swelling in my right thumb came first. Then my second knuckle."

"And the weight loss?" I scribbled notes on my sheet of paper, developing a timeline.

"Hard to say. My weight goes up in the winter, down in the summer. What did your scale say today?"

"238," I said.

"That's low. Wintertime I usually top out at 255, sometimes 260. Bowels looser than usual lately, but I go through that sometimes too. Got a nervous stomach."

"Anything else?"

"Muscle aches. My strength is gone. One night I took my temperature and it was just over 101 degrees. The whole deal is getting me down."

Knowing that I was already 45 minutes behind in my schedule and Joanne had already roomed my next patient, I began to combine questions with the physical exam, beginning with palpation of his neck for thyroid or lymph node enlargement. In assessing whether lymph nodes are abnormal, I gauge whether they are larger than the fingernail on my ring finger, have a rubbery consistency, or are attached to the adjacent soft tissue. Each of these findings suggests a possible malignancy or infection. Leon's lymph nodes were a little generous in size but were not suspicious for cancer.

I asked him to open his mouth. The acrid smell of dental decay was present. Most of his teeth were missing and the rest were rotten and loose. I placed the stethoscope firmly on his upper chest to dampen the background scratching noise chest hair makes. A murmur was present. I motioned the resident over and had her listen.

"Cardiologist told me I have two cusps on the aortic valve instead of three," Leon said. "Told me not to worry about it so I don't." I'd forgotten about the Times crossword puzzle. The man was a sponge for medical jargon.

"Any new sexual partners?" Dr. Litmus asked.

Leon frowned. For a moment there was silence. Then, "My pecker has gone on strike. Not much to say there."

"I'm sorry." The comment by the resident hung for a long moment in the air.

"Me too," Leon shrugged.

Inwardly, I smiled. It was such an innocent, empathetic remark. Truly, here was a doctor in the making whom patients could share their most intimate concerns. "Any shortness of breath? New cough?" I asked, moving on to the lungs.

"Nah, nothing but me and my chronic smoker's cough. I clear out the crud first thing in the morning, then I'm good to go for the rest of the day."

I heard a faint wheeze in the right lung but not in the left. The liver, chronically infected with hepatitis C, was surprisingly normal to palpation. Leon winced slightly when I flexed and extended the left knee. "Orthopedics says I can get a new knee anytime I'm ready. The inner part is bone against bone. If you've got time, I could use a cortisone shot. Seems to hold me for four or five months."

"Sure," I replied. "Let me have Joanne come in and set up for that and I'll be back in a few minutes." The internal medicine resident and I walked back to my office. "Well?" I asked, "Did you get a chance to review the lab?"

"I did. Most of it was abnormal."

"And? What do you think? Want to give me the top four in your differential diagnosis?"

Dr. Litmus cleared her throat and plowed ahead. "Okay. I think he has more than one diagnosis. The knee is a mechanically damaged joint, and the cortisone shot should help, at least for now."

"Okay, I'll give you that. And osteoarthritis probably explains his back pain as well, right? But he has a whole lot going on besides osteoarthritis. Go on."

"Well, the fingers are swollen and stiff, and he has a borderline positive rheumatoid factor in his blood. I've read that sometimes patients with rheumatoid arthritis can have fevers as well as fatigue."

"True," I replied. "Maybe he has RA but it's more or less restricted to his right hand and RA is usually symmetric. Think about his other symptoms: muscle aches, loose bowels, weight loss, sweats. Those are usually outside the spectrum of rheumatoid arthritis. Any other thoughts?

"Smoker. Chronic cough. If he hasn't had a chest X-ray lately that would be on my check-list."

"Good. I'm glad you're widening your thought process beyond classical rheumatology. Lung cancer can sometimes trigger immune inflammation with swollen joints and fevers. So, a chest x-ray would be number one on Willy Sutton's list."

"Willy Sutton?" she asked, raising an eyebrow.

"The bank robber," I answered. "Someone asked him why he robbed banks, and Willie said, 'That's where the money is.' Chest X-ray, good thought."

"But if the chest X-ray is clean," the resident added, "I keep thinking this guy smells like AIDS from shooting up heroin or an old sexual partner. He's losing weight, lymph nodes are a little on the juicy side."

"Testing for AIDS [which, frankly, hadn't crossed my mind] is a great idea," I agreed. "But let's say that his chest X-ray is normal and his HIV test is negative, I'm going to add some rarer disorders, hepatitis C vasculitis and hemochromatosis, to the list."

"Of course!" Dr. Litmus was so excited she could barely contain herself. "That is *so* cool! She looked up and to the right, as if she were channeling a textbook. "To rule out hepatitis C vasculitis, we should pick up cryoglobulins...and hemochromatosis is a genetic disease where we absorb too much iron. It can trigger arthritis and impotence. Leon *has* to have vasculitis or iron overload. Awesome!"

Only he didn't. The chest X-ray and specialized tests were all unremarkable. At our follow-up visit, Leon's joint swelling had spread to the other hand and he'd lost another three pounds. The poor guy could barely make a fist or wipe himself after toileting so I began daily prednisone, telling him that between the positive rheumatoid factor and the symmetry of inflammation, his illness most likely represented rheumatoid arthritis.

"Most likely rheumatoid arthritis?" Leon asked.

"I'm not absolutely certain, but sometimes RA can trigger fevers and weight loss. Low-dose prednisone should help with the pain and swelling while I look into other possibilities." Leon took the prescription and when I called him a week later, he was about 60% better. But the diagnosis didn't sit well with me, like I was trying to cram the diagnosis of RA into a pair of shoes two sizes too small.

When I ran into Dr. Litmus at the hospital several weeks after she finished her rheumatology rotation, she remembered the pig farmer. I reviewed his partial response to prednisone and my tentative diagnosis of rheumatoid arthritis.

"Tentative diagnosis?" she asked. I admitted I wasn't sure, and mentioned that he was still having episodic fevers. She did that odd up-and-out gaze to the right I'd noticed before. "Blood cultures?" she asked. "It's funny how a case can stick with you. The guy had horrible teeth. Maybe a bacterium from an infected tooth got into his circulation and infected his heart valve."

"Good thought," I answered, "but the blood cultures I drew several weeks ago were sterile."

I referred Leon to an infectious disease consultant. Additional tests were dutifully ordered; all of them were unremarkable. Thank goodness the malaria smear was negative, I thought. For a homebody who had never traveled outside the United States, the only way Leon could have developed malaria in Maine would have been if an infected mosquito had snuck into a plane in Africa, been flushed alive down the plane's toilet, and the toilet contents released as the plane passed overhead, misting Leon's pig farm as he came out of the barn.

Leon was a no-show for his next appointment, and the next. I scheduled him for CT scans of his chest and abdomen but he canceled the tests. I called him at home. He reluctantly agreed to the tests. These were unremarkable. At a follow-up visit, he was down another 15 pounds. He groaned as he eased himself into the exam chair.

"Think I got cancer, Doc?" he asked.

I met his eyes. "If you do, I can't find it; the CT scans of your chest and abdomen were normal. I want to arrange for a second opinion at the Massachusetts General Hospital in Boston. Although you may well have rheumatoid arthritis, this is not the usual presentation."

"Boston's out. I've got a sick mother I'm living with on the farm and can't leave her overnight. But hey, at least I can wipe my butt. Had to let my driveway pavement business go."

"Then I'm referring you to hematology. You're anemic and sometimes unusual causes of anemia can only be diagnosed by taking a sample of your bone marrow."

"Let's go for it. I'm no good this way." Hematology initially balked at performing a bone marrow, but when I described Leon's wasting illness, they reluctantly agreed.

The bone marrow was normal.

Leon's weight dipped below 190 pounds. His face developed a pasty, droopy quality. For a man who once weighed 260 pounds, he was beginning to look like photos of Abraham Lincoln. I reluctantly increased his dose of prednisone and added a second rheumatoid arthritis medication. A neighbor helped Leon split and stack two cords of wood. Another neighbor helped him load a truckload of pigs for the slaughterhouse.

During the next month, I found myself drifting back to Leon's case at odd times: on my boat traveling across the bay to Peaks Island; during a hot shower trying to relax before bed, and on first awakening, a vague uneasiness receding into the shadows. I brought up his case at Rheumatology Grand Rounds and my partners suggested additional laboratory testing. These tests were dutifully ordered, but unremarkable.

After a while Leon got tired of coming to see me. Despite his damaged liver, I suspected he'd said to hell with it, and gone back to heavy drinking, maybe even reconnected with his old buddies from his heroin days. I checked the obituaries. Maybe, I thought, he's dead.

Most days, I forgot about Leon. That is, until I was forced to slow down and reflect on my failures. Running across Casco Bay in SAKAMO with the season's first snowstorm, I had plenty of time to ruminate when I ran out of gas midway to Peaks Island. I dropped anchor and called Sea Tow on the marine radio only to hear that it would be more than an hour before they could refuel me. Leon's case rewound in my mind as I rocked on anchor. There was no epiphany.

One day in January—five months after our initial visit, I received a call for a consultation at Maine Medical Center. Leon had been admitted through the ER four days previously with shortness of breath and fevers. He continued to spike fevers despite intravenous antibiotics. Could I come by and take a look at him?

All through morning office hours, my mind kept returning to Leon's case. When my last patient of the morning was a no-show, I decided to visit Leon over lunch. My first stop was radiology in the basement at Maine Medical Center. In the faint white glow of the view box, a chest X-ray from the emergency room showed why he couldn't breathe; the right side of his lung was half-filled with fluid. After reviewing the chest x-ray, the radiologist walked me through the recent abdominal and chest CT scans.

"What's that?" I pointed to a hazy patch adjacent to the chest beneath the right shoulder.

"Lymph node biopsy site." The radiologist turned his head towards me, his pale face glowing eerily in the backlight. "Must be cancer."

I trudged down the hall to pathology. The biopsy results should be ready. After all these months, it made sense that Leon had cancer. It wouldn't be my first time that a cancer mimicked RA or another autoimmune disorder. At least we have tissue, I thought. Maybe it's something treatable. Pathologist Art Vanderburgh located the lymph node biopsy slides and we sat down at a double-headed teaching microscope. "It's an intense inflammatory reaction." He finally said. "No signs of infection or malignancy."

"No signs of cancer cells? Seriously?" I asked. "No cancer?"

Dr. Vanderburgh looked at me sullenly, stone-faced. "I'm a pathologist. Seriously, there is no cancer."

Up on the floor, before examining Leon, I cracked open his chart and reviewed his workup. The admitting team was covering the bases. Assuming that infection was present, Leon had received his first dose of antibiotics in the emergency room. Fluid had been drained from his chest, and blood and urine cultures collected. But he wasn't responding and his fever continued to spike.

When I cracked open the door to Leon's room it was clear he was dying. On the front of the chart was the simple statement: NO CODE. I disengaged emotionally as I stood silently at his bedside, reviewing his case. In another day or two, he'll carry his secret to the grave. Perhaps his mother will sign a permit for an autopsy. Under the methodical scalpel of the pathologist, an autopsy might finally clarify his diagnosis.

Leon's eyes were closed and I reached over and patted his wrist before whispering in his ear, "Keep fighting, Leon. Don't let go."

His nurse entered the room and checked the rate of his IV infusion. I asked if she could call the laboratory and have them draw a red top tube and spin it down and set it aside for me. I pulled out my notebook from my shirt pocket and wrote: *Dont forget to pick up Leon's red top tube.* It will join a half-dozen mystery tubes in my office freezer, awaiting the day when a new case report draws my attention and I draw off an aliquot of fluid for the laboratory to run a newly developed test. Someday, I may know what killed Leon.

Even as I accepted that I did not know the diagnosis, that I might never know Leon's diagnosis, my mind continued to sift through the evidence. It's not cancer. There is no clear evidence for infection. An atypical presentation of one of my diseases? Maybe. He's clearly dying; maybe I should order a pulse dose of steroids? There is an old saying in rheumatology: No one goes to the grave with an undiagnosed disease without a wallop of steroids. Hey, at this point what harm will that do? I clicked my pen and wrote the order*: 1,000 mg intravenous Solu-Medrol. Infuse now*.

Leon shifted his head on the pillow and groaned. His eyes flickered open and settled on me. The faintest whiff of fresh manure permeated the room. Pig farmer. Inflammatory arthritis. Weight loss. Fevers. I cocked my head and clicked my neck. Hepatitis C, diarrhea. Fluid around the heart and lungs. We've looked everywhere for an infection. Maybe it's infection and he's not on the right antibiotic? Maybe it's immunologic and he needs pulse steroids?

My pen hovered over the pulse steroid order. Sign it, notify the medicine team, get it hung, hope for a response. A simple question came to mind. It came from, where? Why not Whipple's disease? Momentarily, I could recall almost nothing about Whipple's disease. Even during my two-year fellowship at Presbyterian University Hospital in Pittsburgh, I'd never encountered a patient with Whipple's. Then I remembered, hadn't I seen it on an extended list of rare causes of diarrhea, weight loss, and inflammatory arthritis? I crossed the steroid order off, closed the chart, and jogged upstairs to the medical library.

Cracking open a rheumatology text I reviewed what little was known about the disease. At the time the article was written, there were only 300 or so cases reported in the world's literature. I learned that the cause of Whipple's disease is a bacterium, *T. whipplei.* Over time, in untreated cases, the infection spreads to lymph nodes and other organs. Arthritis, mimicking rheumatoid arthritis, may be present. In late cases, it spreads to the brain.

The bacteria cannot be cultured. But the organism can be seen on biopsy if the proper stain is applied to the biopsy material. My eyes settled on the last paragraph. *Untreated, the disease is usually fatal. The disease may be more common in workers exposed to manure or raw sewage. Treatment with corticosteroids is generally ineffective. The infection is resistant to many antibiotics but long-term treatment with trimethoprim/sulfasalazine (Bactrim) is usually curative.*

I closed the text and called pathology. No, the biopsy material hadn't been stained for Whipple's disease. Yes, they could stain additional lymph tissue. The slides should be ready tomorrow morning. For the first time in 7 months, I felt confident in my opinion. The shoes fit. It had to be Whipple's disease.

I called the attending on the case. He was reluctant to discontinue the current antibiotic. I had no direct evidence this was Whipple's and was reminded that the current combination of IV antibiotics was usually superior to the older drug Bactrim for a wide variety of infections. Yes, I agreed, but in the case of Whipple's disease, Bactrim was the drug of choice.

Leon's doctor was unconvinced. "Are you sure you don't want to give him a megadose of IV steroids?" he asked.

"No, but do me a favor. If you don't want to stop the current antibiotics, add IV Bactrim tonight. If after restaining the biopsy material pathology doesn't see evidence for Whipple's disease tomorrow, we can stop the Bactrim and I'll order the IV steroids."

The next morning, after a second dose of Bactrim, Leon's fever broke. Art Vanderburgh, the taciturn pathologist, called and wanted me to take a look at the newly stained slides. On slide after slide, *T. whipplei* was present. We marveled at how the organism, now so obvious, could have remained hidden so long.

And ever so slowly, Leon made headway. His arthritis melted away and the diarrhea resolved. Follow-up scans showed that the fluid around his heart and lungs was in full retreat. When his oxygen was discontinued one week later, Leon passed his nurse on the way to the elevator and walked outside to smoke a cigarette. He'd had enough of hospitals. He was a changed man, but not that changed.

We call them zebras: rare diseases hiding in plain sight. They are the great imposters, mimicking everyday infections, cancer, or autoimmune disease. On the day I discharged Leon, the laboratory handed me the extra red top tube of spun-down blood I'd requested. As a mystery solved, I decided to give it to Leon who appreciated the fact that he was still alive. I wrote out the name of the bacteria causing Whipple's disease on the tube. "You never know," he informed me, "when *Tropheryema whipplei* might appear in a Times crossword puzzle."

We both agreed we'd never forget the spelling. I know he won't.

Postscript

Six months later, Leon limped down the hallway at Rheumatology Associates. His beard extended to the middle of his chest and on his feet were the same disheveled gum boots he wore at our first office visit. He had gained back 40 pounds since his hospitalization. At the crook of his elbow was the New York Times crossword puzzle.

On the long-term antibiotic Bactrim, he had made a complete recovery. Considering that he still had a bum knee, a chronic smoker's cough, and a bad back, he felt just fine. His mother had died recently and left him the pig farm. Needless to say, after all he'd been through—Leon was no friend of pigs—he promptly sold it. With the sale of the farm, he bought a motorcycle repair shop. At the conclusion of the visit, Leon stood and shook my hand. "Can the Whipple's come back?"

"I think that's unlikely. Most cases don't relapse, but never say never. We'll see you back in four months and repeat some blood work."

"I'll do that." He pulled a Mason jar of amber-colored honey from his wool jacket and held it up to the light. "I have a few hives on the back lot. It's been a good year for honey. You know," he continued, "there's a hell of a lot to keep track of in apiculture. And what's more, the word apiculture is a favorite of cruciverbalists." He handed me the honey jar. I never saw him again.

Chapter 7

"This disease was on the verge of being discovered. Somebody had to do it." F. Wagner 1940

In my rheumatology practice, I am on-call for one week every six weeks. My friends, who have a peripheral knowledge of rheumatology, gently poke fun at me when I remind them that I'm on-call and can't go hiking or travel too far afield. Example e-mail: *Disappointed you can't hike Mount Washington. Emergency! Stat! You must rush to hospital! Inflamed joint!* And of course, it *is* true that rheumatology usually lacks the pivotal life and death decisions of neurosurgery or cardiology or emergency medicine.

Even so, my week on call is packed with both the mundane and the unexpected, and yes, the occasional emergency. It's my turn to see hospital consultations for the group, review patients' labs and X-rays for my partners who are out of the office, answer phone calls from primary care providers looking for curbside consults—and this is where I most enjoy life as a rheumatologist—I fit in sick patients with unknown suspected immunologic disorders.

So, it was not out of the ordinary when I opened a chart outside an exam room one blustery winter evening and reviewed an unusual story. The patient, Mrs. Shones, age fifty-six, had been sick for three months. Previously healthy, she had developed a nagging sinus infection, or at least what appeared to be a sinus infection. A month later a painful right ear brought her back to her family doctor and she was diagnosed with a middle ear infection. When she didn't improve on multiple antibiotics, she was referred to an ear-nose-and-throat specialist (ENT) who placed a tube in the ear to facilitate drainage, and this worked, for a while. That is, until the opposite ear became painful.

ENT was perplexed and referred her to an allergist. But the workup for allergies was negative, and intermittent fevers settled in. A course of prednisone was empirically prescribed (definition of empirically prescribed: *I don't know what's wrong but let's try a course of prednisone)*. The fluid resolved and the fevers transiently improved, but then relapsed off prednisone. An infectious disease specialist was consulted to assess whether an unusual infection might be behind her bouts of sinusitis. Despite extensive testing, nothing was found.

So far, I thought to myself, I'm not sure if this is relevant as to why I'm seeing Mrs.…I flipped the chart back to the front, Mrs. Shones. I felt a tug at my elbow. Joanne whispered, "Phone call. It's Dr. Miller [one of my partners in my rheumatology practice]. He's at Maine Medical Center and wants to sign out a hospital consult."

I glanced into the exam room of my new patient. She was seated, her hands covering her face, and sobbing. I scratched my ear, uncertain what to say and stepped inside. "Are you okay?"

Mrs. Shones lifted her head and massaged her forehead. Her blouse was soaked in sweat and the bridge of her nose was reddened and swollen like a boxer's. I noticed that the left side of her face drooped like soft clay. I asked myself: *Why is this woman in my office instead of the emergency room?*

"I have a terrible headache," she whispered. The last few weeks, my muscles and joints have been killing me. I feel like I've been kicked by a mule." She massaged her forehead and coughed. "May I lie down?"

"Of course. Here, let me..." I helped her onto the exam table.

Joanne called from the doorway, "Should I tell Dr. Miller to call back?"

"Go on," Mrs. Shones insisted. "I've had the paralysis on the left side of my face for weeks. My doctor calls it Bell's palsy. The fevers and sweats come every evening, but this..." she rolled up a pant leg. "This is new. I woke up with it several days ago." The calf was peppered with red spots ranging in size from a single dot to the size of a quarter. "You're just happening to see me at my worst. I'll be fine, go on and take your call."

I asked Joanne to remain with Mrs. Shones and to repeat her blood pressure. On my way to my office, the laboratory supervisor caught up with me. "Does your new consult need blood drawn?" Which was code for: *It's 6:30 on a Friday night. Can I close the lab and go home?*

"Sorry, but I need a CBC and basic chemistries stat. Sick lady." I briefly considered Mrs. Shones's bare-bone history and her dramatic physical findings and scribbled down a laundry list of laboratory studies. "I think this will do it. Looks like it's starting to snow. I'll close up the building after the results are printed out. Have a safe drive home."

Returning to my office I picked up the phone. "Dr. Miller, what do you have for me?"

"One more patient for you to see over the weekend. I just tapped a hot, swollen knee in 335b at Maine Medical Center, and I'm on my way down to the laboratory to check the fluid. Probably gout, but could be infection. I'll leave a note on the chart summarizing the results. Big guy, I mean BIG guy, had to use a spinal needle to get fluid. Felt like I was drilling for oil and hit a gusher. I drew off 80 cc of fluid and..."

"Dr' Radis," Joanne's voice carried down the hallway. "We need your help. Now."

I hung up the phone and jogged back to Mrs. Shones's room, pushed open the door, and...blood was splattered everywhere. Joanne held Mrs. Shones upright, a plastic basin pressed up against her mouth. A look of absolute horror was frozen on both their faces. Mrs. Shones tried to stifle another cough, swallowed, and swallowed again. Like an exorcism gone horribly wrong, she wretched, and blood shot out of her mouth.

I picked up the phone and called 911 as Joanne ran for our oxygen tank.

Minutes later, an ambulance rolled to a stop at the back entrance and I helped load Mrs. Shones onto a gurney. As the ambulance raced up Congress Street to Maine Medical Center, I followed in my Jeep and parked on a side street, a block away from the emergency room. Slogging my way towards the ER entrance through four inches of fresh snow, I recalled the marine forecast: light winds from the north, poor visibility, with six to eight inches of additional snow.

My flip phone vibrated. It was the laboratory technician. "Dr. Radis? I have the results for your last patient. It's a mess. I remember my grandmother when she was this anemic. She needed a blood transfusion! Did your lady go home?"

"That's a negative, and I think a transfusion is clearly in her future. Anything else?"

"Yes. It's all bad." He rattled off the numbers. "Her level of inflammation, the CRP, is through the roof. Any idea why she'd be in kidney failure?"

"We're trying to sort that out," I replied. "Thanks for staying late. I really appreciate it. This information is going to be very helpful." The differential diagnosis had dramatically shifted in the past fifteen minutes. The skin rash was almost certainly vasculitis, and vasculitis was one of my diseases. Mrs. Shones was in the correct office after all.

As I passed through the ER sliding doors, I preemptively removed a stethoscope from my soft briefcase, draped it around my neck and ran a hand through my hair. Although I was on staff at Maine Medical Center, this was not my community hospital across town where I was well known. Without the customary thigh-length white coat most attending physicians wore, I knew that my identity could be challenged. I flipped through my wallet looking for my rarely used medical staff ID card. *Hmm, I wonder where that could be....*

The charge nurse was closing in, "Can I help you?" Code for: *exactly who are you and why are you standing at my nursing station?*

I took her hand in mine and said that it was a pleasure to meet her. "Dr. Radis, rheumatology. My patient, Mrs. Shones, just came in by ambulance. What room is she in?"

"And do you have any..."

"Who's the attending on her case? I have some laboratory results and clinical information which might help clarify her diagnosis."

The charge nurse reluctantly handed me the chart. "Mrs. Shones is in cubicle #3. Dr. Smith is the attending. She ordered a stat CBC, type and crossed-matched her for four units of blood, and a portable chest X-ray. The bleeding has stopped. We're all set."

"And her chest X-ray?" I asked. "Will the X-ray technician hang the films over there?" I pointed to the back wall.

"Yes," the charge nurse's tone suggested that I was both irrelevant and mildly irritating.

"Great." I surreptitiously pulled out my pocket planner and scribbled, *Keep Maine Medical Center ID badge in satchel.*

I sat down to review Dr. Smith's note. Across from me was a vaguely familiar internal medicine resident. Her blue scrubs were bloodstained around the ankles; her eyes drooped nearly shut. For the first time, I noticed that my own shoes and socks were soaked in blood. The X-ray technician hung Mrs. Shones's chest X-ray on the screen behind us and I slowly exhaled. The outline of the heart was the only normal finding. White irregular patches obscured both lower lung fields. Four nodules, one the size of a golf ball, were clearly visible in the mid and upper lungs. "Vasculitis," I whispered to myself.

Dr. Smith emerged from Mrs. Shones's room and strode over to the view box. She turned towards the internal medicine resident and pointed out the nodules. "This most likely represents metastatic disease to the lung. Poor thing, one of the tumors must have eroded into a blood vessel and triggered the bleeding. In her age group, metastatic breast cancer is the most likely diagnosis. Admit her to the ICU. Call pulmonary medicine. If there's no known primary, they may need to scope her to make a diagnosis. If it's not cancer, maybe multiple lung abscesses from infection."

The internal medicine resident's eyes sharpened as she scanned the chest X-ray. "Could it be vasculitis?"

"Vasculitis?" Dr. Smith tipped her head and restudied the chest X-ray. "Well, vasculitis can mimic a lot of diseases, so sure, I guess we can add that to the list. Cathy," she called out to the charge nurse, "can you hang that first unit of blood for Shones as soon as it comes up from the blood bank?" She looked up at the patient board, multitasking, already on to her next patient evaluation. Dr. Smith's job was done.

"Dr. Smith," I caught up to her and extended my hand as she was about to duck into another cubicle. "Chuck Radis, rheumatology. I was consulting on Mrs. Shones tonight at the office when she began to cough up blood and I called for the ambulance. Did you get a chance to roll up her slacks and take a look at her legs? I think she has…"

"No, not yet. As you can see, we're kind of busy here tonight. Packed. I'll pass it on to the team." She turned away.

"Dr. Smith, I need to show you something. It'll take only a moment." I pulled back the curtain to the cubicle. Mrs. Shones was curled onto her side in a fetal position, unresponsive, her oxygen mask in a pool of blood on the floor. Instinctively, Dr. Smith pulled the code cart into the room. Respiratory therapy suctioned blood from Mrs. Shones's mouth and placed a fresh oxygen mask on her face. Nursing handed Dr. Smith a mask and helped her into a pair of sterile gloves—in case this was an unusual infection such as tuberculosis or HIV.

I stood off to the side.

A thready pulse was present. Management of her vasculitis, though it was the root cause of her illness, would need to wait. Dr. Smith quickly lowered the head of the stretcher and inserted a laryngoscope into the patient's mouth to visualize the vocal cords, just as Mrs. Shones coughed again and blood obscured the airway. Respiratory therapy gently applied suction.

"Give me more suction! Clear out the back of the throat!" In her left hand she held the laryngoscope steady. In her right was the endotracheal tube. "Stay to the left of the midline with the suction. Give me a shot at the cords! That's it." She slid the tube through the vocal cords. Dr. Smith exhaled. We all exhaled. Minutes later Mrs. Shones was on her way to the intensive care unit. I drifted down to the cafeteria for a cup of coffee. I'll give the ICU team time to settle Mrs. Shone in before I introduce myself to the team.

In the world of rare diseases, vasculitis is a broad and complex topic. The definition is simple enough: vasculitis refers to any condition which triggers inflammation and damage to a blood vessel. Downstream blood flow is reduced, or in many cases, completely blocked. Depending on the distribution of vasculitis and the size of the blood vessels involved, the results may be catastrophic: kidney failure, lung hemorrhage, stroke, death.

In some forms of vasculitis, the triggers are well known. The HIV virus may trigger vasculitis in AIDS patients. Vasculitis is associated with both the hepatitis B and C viruses. Several prescription medications may rarely trigger vasculitis. But there are mysterious vasculitis syndromes whose triggers remain unknown. These life-threatening disorders often settle onto patients like a slow-acting poison. In their earliest stage, they mimic common disorders: headaches, sinus or middle ear infections, or chronic headaches. And because a medical practitioner may go an entire practice lifetime without seeing a case of vasculitis, the diagnosis is often missed or delayed, particularly if early on the skin is spared.

Cup of coffee in hand, I clicked open the door to the ICU. At the nursing station, I spotted the same internal medicine resident I had briefly seen in the ER. It was Dr. Litmus. Slumped over a chart, her hair pulled back in a haphazard bun, she was nearly unrecognizable. I tapped her on the shoulder and asked if she was admitting Mrs. Shones. "Shones?" she replied wearily as she scanned her list of recent admissions. "I just finished. Seriously, I know the case but forgot the name. It's been 36 hours since I've been off call; I'm pinch-hitting for my friend who's pregnant and is on her ICU rotation. Hey! I heard that the pig farmer with the fevers and weight loss we saw together in the office ended up having Whipple's disease! That is *so* cool! Is he okay?"

It was my turn to smile. I had heard through a colleague that UCLA had accepted Dr. Litmus for a cardiology fellowship but as yet, she hadn't accepted the position. There was still a slim chance she might change her mind and go into rheumatology. "You wouldn't recognize him," I said. "He's gained back all of his weight. Next time I see him in the office, I'll tell him you asked about him. So…what's up with Mrs. Shones?"

"In the dumpster, really sick. Her kidneys have shut down. Pulmonary says she's too unstable to undergo bronchoscopy, so we can't get a biopsy of the lung nodules. Even on the ventilator, she's barely hanging on. Oh! I completely forgot. I heard you saw her earlier tonight in the office. Did you see her lower legs? They're peppered with a blotchy red rash. I ran up to the library and opened a dermatology text and it looks like a condition called *palpable purpura*. Could she have vasculitis?"

"Yes. Absolutely. Are you sure you don't want to go into rheumatology?"

At the bedside we pulled back the sheets and silently assessed the rash. Several of the lesions were ulcerated, exposing the deeper salmon-colored fatty tissues adjacent to the calf muscles. I silently reviewed where we stood and worked my way back from the known to the unknown. As I recalled the history, it wasn't until prednisone, a potent anti-inflammatory, was prescribed for the persistent swelling in the middle ear that Mrs. Shones transiently improved. And the rest, the muscle and joint aches, the cough and facial droop, the lung nodules, were undoubtedly all part of one disease process. We were in the final stages of a fulminating, deadly vasculitis.

It had to be *granulomatosis* with *polyangiitis*, or GPA.

GPA is a horrendous disease. Prior to 1950, almost no one survived beyond six months. High-dose prednisone lengthened the average life-expectancy of GPA sufferers to 18 months, but did not change the outcome: with few exceptions, the diagnosis was a death sentence. And death often came with horrific suffering.

It was not until the chemotherapy drug Cytoxan was given to patients in the late 1970s that patients could reasonably hope for a long-term remission, or in some cases, a cure. For that, we have Dr. Anthony Fauci and his colleagues at the National Institute of Health to thank. By borrowing Cytoxan from the world of cancer medicine, Fauci established a new standard of care in the management of life-threatening vasculitis.

From my briefcase I took out a skin biopsy kit, sterilized the right calf with an antiseptic, and obtained a sample of the involved skin. In a sick, unstable patient like Mrs. Shones, the skin is often the only area where we can safely confirm the diagnosis of vasculitis. Definitive proof of *GPA* will rely on the presence of an ANCA (short for: anti-neutrophil cytoplasmic antibody) in a blood sample. One problem: The blood test is sent to the Massachusetts General Hospital's immunology laboratory and the result will take up to a week to return. We don't have the luxury of waiting. Treatment will need to be initiated before we can confirm the diagnosis of GPA.

I huddled at the nursing station with Paul Parker, MD, the kidney specialist on the case. He'd already noted the lower leg rash and strongly suspected GPA. In addition to my plan for high-dose steroids and the chemotherapy drug Cytoxan, he suggested that we add plasmapheresis. Technically, plasmapheresis involves removing antibodies from the blood through a process similar to hemodialysis, and then adding back donated plasma. In simple terms, plasmapheresis is in with the good and out with the bad, a complex reworking of the Greek concept of balancing the four body humors. And it works, sometimes.

After finishing my note I took the elevator downstairs, zipped up my parka, and waded through calf-deep snow on the way to my Jeep. I glanced at my watch. I should have plenty of time to park the Jeep at the ferry terminal and easily make the last ferry to Peaks Island. Keys in hand, I wandered up and down the darkened street several times searching for the Jeep. A hospital security guard sauntered over. "Parking ban tonight. I saw a tow truck out here 15 minutes ago. Your Jeep?"

I half-closed my eyes. "Unfortunately, yes." I was bone tired. I felt like sitting down in the snow. "I'm trying to make the 10:30 ferry back to Peaks Island."

The policeman eyed me sympathetically. "You know, if you hurry, you might have time to jog to the outdoor parking lot on Franklin Street where they towed your Jeep, pay your fine, and make the last ferry. It's what, maybe a mile?" He leaned in so I could see his face and smiled. "Dr. Radis, you don't recognize me, do you?"

I squinted back in the dim light. "Bob? Broadway Bob?"

"You got it!" He snapped his fingers. "Island Services. It's been a few years, but I used to take you out to the outer islands for house calls in the police boat. Listen, I can't leave my beat, but I think you can make the ferry if you hurry. By the way, you've got blood on your shoes and pant leg."

I glanced down. "It's a long story," I shrugged. "Thanks for the information." Then I took off down the hill, slip-sliding in the fresh snow. Turning right on Park Street, I picked up the pace, my wool hat pulled down over my eyes against the biting wind. Then a gust of wind peeled the wool cap off my head and it tumbled behind me in the snow. Just ahead, I could see the brightly lit parking lot. There was my Jeep, the only vehicle in the empty lot, the first to be towed in the entire city.

Out of the corner of my eye I spied a tow truck turn into the lot with another vehicle and a figure emerge from a nearby booth. I jogged over, and pointing to my watch, desperately pleaded my case. "That's my Jeep over there! Fourteen minutes! I only have fourteen minutes before the last ferry leaves for Peaks Island!"

The attendant looked up from his clipboard and did a double take. A delicate layer of snow covered my head. Ice encrusted my mustache and eyebrows. My parka was thrown open; my pants caked in snow where I had fallen coming into the lot. Never mind the bloody shoes. He held out the clipboard. "Fifty bucks. Cash. Sign here. Your keys are in the booth."

After paying the fine, I jumped into the Jeep and fishtailed out of the lot, only to lightly press on the brakes coming to the first red light. Careful. Don't be an idiot. I waited for the light to change and then abruptly relaxed. Too late. As the saying goes: If you're not on the boat, you're off the boat. The ferry *always* leaves on time.

Of course, there was always SAKAMO. Coming out of the parking lot I looked across to the adjacent wharf and there she was, bobbing on her lines. With the snow, the visibility on the water will be reduced. I'll need to navigate by compass. But hey, the wind has dropped off. What could possibly go wrong?

After shoveling out the boat, I motored due east until I passed Spring Point Ledge Lighthouse, then pointed the bow towards a barely visible red blinking light marking the shallow water off House Island. Abruptly, less than a half mile from my dock on Peaks Island, SAKAMO shuddered to a stop. I shut off the engine and checked the fuel tank. Full. I turned on the VHF marine radio and verified that it was fully charged if I needed to make an emergency call to the Coast Guard. Then I pressed the hydraulic button on the thruster and tilted the engine out of the water to inspect the propeller. A lobster buoy line was wrapped hopelessly around the propeller shaft. This was not the first time I'd picked up a ghost buoy (a lobster buoy pulled beneath the surface by drifting seaweed).

After snugging up my life preserver, I grabbed a knife from the overhead shelf inside the pilot house and was about to lean over the stern and cut the line when I heard waves breaking nearby. The wind and current were pushing SAKAMO towards the ledges. I turned on the cabin light and located my anchor and flung it overboard. When I was satisfied that the anchor held and I was no longer drifting, I tied one end of a line to a cleat and the other to my life preserver before I leaned out over the stern and cut through the tangled mess on the propeller.

In a few minutes I was underway.

At home, dripping wet in the mudroom, Sandi met me with two hair dryers and gave me a brief hug. "I'm so relieved that you didn't miss the last ferry home. The upstairs pipes are frozen in the bathroom. Can you work the pipes in the downstairs bathroom? We need to unfreeze them before they burst."

I stepped into the brightly lit kitchen and her face drooped. My hands and coat were smeared with grease, my pants an oily, tattered mess. Sandi's critical eye missed the bloody shoes. "What happened? Your clothes are ruined."

"I missed the last ferry and decided to take SAKAMO home. Near House Island I picked up a lobster buoy and had to cut it off the prop." I sat down at the kitchen table, realizing for the first time, just how miserable I really was. "I'm cold. *Really* cold."

"Were you wearing your life preserver?"

"Yes."

"You didn't run out of gas, did you? You promised me that you were going to always keep an extra can of gas onboard."

"No. Plenty of gas."

"Good." Satisfied that I was mostly okay, Sandi's practical side took over. "Let's get you warmed up and into some dry clothes." She opened the oven door and turned on the heat as I peeled off my ruined clothes. Dressed in a spare parka, insulated socks and underwear, a knit hat, and gloves, I slowly unthawed.

Then it was time to get to work, Sandi in the upstairs bathroom, me in our tiny downstairs bathroom. Twenty minutes later we heard the welcome tinkling of slush ice moving through the pipes and took a hot shower together. After drying off, we turned back the faucets to a continuous drip to keep the pipe from refreezing and went to bed.

The next day when I made early morning rounds at Maine Medical Center, Mrs. Shones was still alive. During the night she'd been transfused with six units of blood to stabilize her blood counts. Specialized nurses from the nephrology department stopped by to hook Mrs. Shones up for her second round of plasmapheresis. I wrote the orders for intravenous Cytoxan.

Five days into Mrs. Shones's admission, I received a call at home from Dr. John Niles, a kidney specialist from the Massachusetts General Hospital. After an exhausting week on call, I'd gone to bed early. John wanted to talk about my patient. I swung my legs over the edge of the bed and glanced at the bedside clock. My mind went into hyper-alert. "Dr. Niles, what are you doing in the immunology laboratory this late? Don't you ever go home?"

"Hanging out. Just hanging out. Dr. Radis, I have the results of your ANCA testing on a Mrs. Shones, age fifty-six, and saw your name and phone number on the requisition slip. I'm calling to tell you that it's markedly positive. Classic for GPA. The titer is sky high."

"Sick lady," I answered, grabbing my pen and a loose sheet of paper.

"Can you tell me more about the case?" he asked.

"Five-month history of sinus inflammation, fevers, recent lower extremity ulcerating rash, lung nodules, and kidney failure. The works," I answered. "I saw her in the office last week for the first time and she coughed up a pint of blood, and was intubated within a few hours. We haven't been able to wean her from the ventilator yet."

"Well, I'm not surprised. I haven't seen an ANCA this high for a long time. GPA can smolder for months and then everything goes to hell. Is she on plasmapheresis? Cytoxan? IV steroids?" he asked.

"Yes, all three. Out with the bad humors, in with the good." I couldn't help but grin. It was nine o'clock on a Friday night, and Dr. John Niles, the lead author on numerous medical journal articles on GPA, was on the line and wanted to hear more about a lady in Maine on a ventilator balancing between life and death.

He wondered what dose of Cytoxan I had given Mrs. Shones. After providing him with the numbers, I could hear a pencil scratching out calculations before he declared, "That's a very reasonable dose." I said that she was maybe, a tad better.

When John Niles told me that she was going to be all right, that he'd been in exactly the same spot three weeks ago, and only yesterday discharged that patient home, I felt reassured. John Niles lives and breathes vasculitis. From long experience, he had a sense for where the numbers were headed.

"She's going to be all right," he repeated, before hanging up. "Crazy disease, isn't it? Ten cases per million people per year and we're no closer to figuring out the cause than we were thirty years ago."

"I think you need to work a little harder, John," I suggested.

There was a pause. I wondered how he might react. "That's a joke, isn't it?" he finally replied.

"Yes," I answered, smiling. "And thanks so much for the work you've done on this disease. It's a monster."

Chapter 8

After dark, I picked my way down the gangplank to SAKAMO on the Portland waterfront. Then I grabbed a paddle and fractured the ice, making room for SAKAMO to exit her slip. Even with the last several nights well below zero, I hoped that the bay would be relatively open. That said, it was reassuring when a lobster boat, its deck piled high with traps, its bow bearded in ice, turned into an adjacent slip. The captain leaned out from the pilot house and, recognizing me, shouted, "Stay to the north side of the ship channel. You should be fine."

I hesitated. Just because a 40-foot lobster boat was "fine" coming into port, doesn't mean that I'll avoid a white-knuckle ride home. On the adjacent wharf, the Casco Bay Lines ferry was loading. I jogged over to the ferry, purchased a ticket to Peaks Island, and was the last passenger to board.

Tomorrow, I was leaving for Guatemala on a 10-day medical trip and hoped to arrive home tonight before Kate and Molly went to bed. I settled wearily onto a long bench in the hold of the ferry and wrote in my pocket planner: *DON'T FORGET PASSPORT! Bring medical supplies for joint injections, arthritis medications, stethoscope, two pairs of surgical scrubs. DON'T FORGET*

PASSPORT! I looked over the list with frank pessimism. Perhaps Sandi can double-check my suitcase tonight. Another pair of eyes wouldn't hurt.

This was to be my first medical trip abroad and I was, similar to my youngest daughter Molly's reflection on her first Halloween on Peaks Island, "a little scared and a little happy." While in medical school, I had envisioned taking breaks from my practice to volunteer in high-need communities. This coming week, in my role as a volunteer for a U.S.-based nonprofit, I would evaluate and treat villagers in the shadow of Mt. Fuego, an active volcano.

I snugged up my parka for the fifteen-minute walk home (our truck's battery was dead) and my thoughts drifted back to my last office patient of the day, Mrs. Shones, my *GPA* patient. As Dr. Niles at the Massachusetts General Hospital had predicted, she had survived but with permanent damage to her lungs and kidneys. Even so, she was back working part-time as an editor for a small publishing house, a job she could do from home.

At today's visit she lasered in on two issues. Can I reduce the dose of prednisone? And the nose, what can we do about my nose? During her hospitalization, at the height of her life-threatening inflammation, the cartilage in the bridge of her nose had collapsed. Now the nose sat in the center of her face like a battered pug nose on a boxer's face. With our focus on her survival, the nose, at the time, had seemed like the least of our worries.

Mrs. Shones lightly ran a finger along the sunken cartilage. "I saw the plastic surgeon you referred me to in Boston earlier this week. She says she can implant a graft where the cartilage was destroyed and reconstruct the nose. But first, I need to be on lower-dose prednisone, preferably none, so the tissue can heal properly. Is my GPA ready for that?"

The laboratory tech knocked on the door and handed me two sheets of laboratory results. The numbers continued to slowly improve and I recommended that we decrease the prednisone by another 10 mg. "If all goes well," I said, "you can get the nose fixed by early summer."

Coming in view of our house, I knew that in all likelihood, even with the temperatures in the single digits, the girls would be outside playing in the snow. Sandi shares her mother's parenting style from growing up on the family dairy farm: If you're bored, read a book or go outside and play. If you're cold, snug up your wool hat and wear mittens over a pair gloves. Have fun. Despite the hour, I changed into insulated boots and joined Kate and Molly as they careened down our hill in their plastic sleds. On one hair-raising run, both girls stood on their sleds holding onto the ropes. Off to the north, the faint glow of the northern lights shimmered on the horizon.

A half hour later, we retreated inside, and as the girls peeled off their winter parkas and snow pants, they complained that their hands were cold. I noticed that several fingers on both girls' hands were blanched white from the knuckles to the fingertips, a condition called Raynaud's phenomenon. My stomach churned. Although Raynaud's may occur commonly in children and adults as an isolated condition, it may also be an early sign of an immune system disorder.

The girls were otherwise healthy, but the Raynaud's concerned me. I wondered, with the delicate checks and balances in our immune system, were they only one immunologic misstep away from developing lupus or rheumatoid arthritis? Inside the house, their fingers quickly regained color and I jotted down in my pocket calendar: *Ask pediatrician to draw basic immunology lab on girls.*

My work in Guatemala was, in many ways, a major disappointment. Medications were freely dispensed for painful knees and back injuries. I injected a damaged wrist with cortisone. A Mayan woman in her early 20's stood patiently in line holding the hand of her two-year-old daughter to be evaluated. Through an interpreter, I learned that the mother's fingers, knees, and ankles had been swollen and stiff for more than a year. A diagnosis of rheumatoid arthritis was clear, but the barriers to treatment were formidable. Concerned that she could get pregnant while on methotrexate (which raises the risk of birth defects), I recommended a safer but oftentimes less effective medication in its place and spent the rest of my week trying to connect the woman to a local practitioner. Eventually, I paid up front for six months of medications, office visits, and blood draws.

I felt cautiously optimistic that the woman was in good hands. Three months later however, her doctor emailed me that she was lost to follow-up. Despite my good intentions, I failed to provide the care this woman so sorely needed.

While overseas *surgical* missions undoubtably play a vital role in improving the lives of individuals—for instance, cleft palate surgery or cataract surgery—impacting chronic diseases like diabetes, hypertension, and rheumatoid arthritis is much more challenging and complex. If not funded and coordinated with local healthcare providers, these patients often fall by the wayside. A month or two of free blood pressure medications or a cortisone injection in the knee for rheumatoid arthritis does little to improve long-term health. There was little reason to be proud of my work in Guatemala.

After returning home, I came across a quote from the American author Teju Cole, on the "success" of overseas volunteer medical missions. His characterization of my trip to Guatemala would have been brutally frank. "The White Savior Industrial Complex is not about justice. Medical missions are about a big emotional experience that validates privilege... If we are going to interfere in the lives of others, a little due diligence is a minimum requirement." Harsh, but sadly, in my own experience, an often-true characterization.

It was not until more than a decade later when I volunteered in India that I found a meaningful niche in overseas medical work. My experience at the Bangalore Baptist Hospital, teaching family practice and internal medicine residents the art of rheumatologic diagnosis and treatment, was deeply satisfying. But there were major limitations in the care of patients in this resource-poor setting. While only a small percentage of my patients in Maine progressed to disability due to lack of resources, at the time, this was the general rule in India.

On one particularly heart-wrenching house call in India, I accompanied a young doctor to the home of a woman in her early twenties who spent her days keeping warm on a cot next to the fire. For 10 years her mother had helplessly watched as rheumatoid arthritis ravaged her daughter Maria's shoulders, wrists, knees, and hips. Every morning, the mother picked up her 80-pound daughter from her bed like a package and placed her on the cot.

Despite liberal use of anti-inflammatories and morphine four times daily, Maria groaned continuously during my exam. I asked the Indian doctor if orthopedics would consider joint replacements and his answer was both practical and poignant. "For the cost of a hip or knee replacement, we can immunize more than a thousand children."

When I returned from India, I recounted the story of Maria to my colleagues at my weekly rheumatology conference. Our oldest member, Phil Thompson, MD, reminded us that in the 1960s, "a wing at Maine Medical Center was devoted to patients, some as young as three years old, with rheumatologic disorders. Many of them died at a very young age, either from their diseases, or from complications of treatment. Our failures far outnumbered our successes."

Today, I occasionally consult on "old-time" rheumatoid arthritis patients in my practice, patients whose disease has progressed without the benefit of recent advances in treatment. Or worse, patients who dramatically improve with recent advances in treatment only to have it suddenly discontinued due to lack of insurance or high co-pays.

This reality hit home once again in 2022, when I received a phone call about a family from war-torn Ukraine and their five-year-old daughter, previously diagnosed with juvenile idiopathic arthritis. The family had arrived in Maine with nothing but the clothes they could carry and were taken in by friends on nearby Cliff Island. I spoke with the father who was worried that without his daughter's weekly injection of Humira (begun in Ukraine), her arthritis would relapse and she would soon be confined to a wheelchair. I called my colleague Ed Fels, a pediatric rheumatologist, who arranged for her to restart this critical medication. Today, she continues to do well. No one would suspect that she suffers from childhood arthritis.

But what if the family had landed in a refugee settlement? Or what if the newer medications were simply unaffordable? We should never take for granted the immense progress basic science, clinical trials, and the availability of effective treatment has made in our patients' lives.

Chapter 9

"Healing is impossible without trust. With trust, if you can't cure, you may still heal."
Dr. Abraham Verghese

What struck me first as I walked by the exam room where Lynn P. sat was the swelling in her fingers. Her hands rested unnaturally on her thighs, palms up, the fingers slightly flexed. She had an air of simple straightforward expectation, as if she might hold out her hands and ask if she could have a refund for another better functioning pair.

Outside the room, I picked up the chart and skimmed through the notes her family doctor had forwarded: *Two months postpartum... uncomplicated pregnancy .... healthy 7 lb., 6 oz. boy...breastfeeding, abrupt onset swelling of fingers and wrists.* Next visit: *Swelling and pain persist in fingers, worse in a.m., toesand ankles stiff.* And then: *Trouble holding baby, lab studies okay, but getting worse by the day. Rheumatology referral.*

I turned to the information questionnaire she had filled out: 27 years old, born in Portland, Maine. Second-grade teacher. Married. First pregnancy. No significant past medical history. No surgeries. No allergies. Nonsmoker. I could see where she crossed out her original answer, no alcohol, to *well, I had a glass of wine last week to see if it could help me sleep, but no luck!*

Ever so gingerly, I shook her hand as I entered the room. The wrists and fingers were a boggy swollen mass of inflammation. She limply withdrew her hand and thanked me for seeing her on short notice. Only then did I notice the baby carrier tucked under the table at her feet. She had brought her son.

The mysterious onset of inflammatory arthritis beginning shortly after childbirth has a limited differential diagnosis. Mysterious, in that affected women often have no history of previous health problems, have uncomplicated deliveries, and the baby is completely well. In the usual case, there have been no unusual exposures, no preceding illness. One day the new mother is well, the next her joints begin to stiffen and swell.

I mulled over the possibilities. Despite the absence of the usual signs such as fever or rash, perhaps Lynn P.'s swollen joints were triggered by a viral infection. I recalled that Parvovirus B-19 may be a cause of life-altering arthritis, but that in nearly all cases, the arthritis resolves over weeks to months. Lyme disease? Two recent Lyme tests were negative and Lyme arthritis is usually restricted to one or two large joints, say a knee or wrist. Lupus may present with painful, swollen joints, but as I fleshed out her history and examined her more fully, I was convinced that this was unlikely as well.

Lynn P. held out her hands. On closer inspection, the joints adjacent to the fingernails were uniformly normal, while the middle joints and knuckles were tender and swollen. When I asked her to make a fist, she winced, and could curl the fingers only partway to the palm. Her son stirred and cried out. Lynn held him briefly before gently returning him to the bassinette beneath the chair.

Rheumatologists often arrive at a definitive diagnosis in a decidedly low-tech fashion. The distribution of inflamed joints narrows the possibilities. For instance, swelling of all three joints in a single finger or toe (giving the appearance of a sausage), may be seen in psoriatic arthritis, while the arthritis of Crohn's disease, an immune system disorder affecting the bowel, typically affects larger joints such as the knees or ankles. Rheumatoid arthritis (RA) tends to be symmetric, and early on, frequently inflames the knuckles and middle joints of both hands.

Sliding my hand up the forearm, a fleshy, rubbery nodule the size of a marble was palpable at the bony prominence of each elbow. The growths are so specific for rheumatoid arthritis that they are called rheumatoid nodules. The moment I felt the nodules my mind shifted away from considering a number of possibilities to a firm conclusion. Between the inflammation in her fingers and the nodules at the elbows, Lynn P. almost certainly had rheumatoid arthritis. The difficult work of adjusting to a lifelong inflammatory disease lay before her.

I silently reviewed the lab Lynn's doctor had enclosed. It's not that laboratory testing is irrelevant in rheumatology, it's that both positive and negative results need to be interpreted carefully. For example, her rheumatoid factor blood test was negative, but one in five RA patients are never positive for tests linked to RA. What's more, the opposite is also true. A positive rheumatoid factor does not always indicate RA. It can also be seen in viral infections, tuberculosis, and in families with a history of rheumatoid arthritis.

Although I was nearly certain of the diagnosis of rheumatoid arthritis, I hesitated. Lynn P. had volunteered almost nothing besides simple yes and no answers to my questions. There was a degree of coolness on her part, as if she were holding me at arm's length. As she reached down beneath her chair and quietly rocked the bassinet, I realized I had no sense of who she was beyond the bare bones of her office questionnaire.

Even so, rather than inquiring about her baby or recent experiencesas a second-grade teacher, I decided it was time to tell her what I thought was wrong. This was my first mistake. I could have made a therapeutic connection, hedged, ordered additional laboratory testing, and seen her back in one week. Instead, I closed the chart and asked, "Have you noticed the bumps at the back of your elbows?"

Lynn P. pressed each nodule between her thumb and index finger and looked at me blankly. "They're called rheumatoid nodules," I continued. "Unfortunately, between the joint inflammation in your hands, and the rheumatoid nodules at the elbows, I'm sorry to say, you have early rheumatoid arthritis." I paused. Questions? Shock? Disbelief? Nothing. I took out a colored pen and sketched a diagram of a finger joint.

"If we work our way from the outside to the inside of a joint, we first come across the capsule. This is the substance that firmly holds a joint together. Picture the last time you ate chicken wings and perhaps you noticed the shiny tough substance connecting one part of the 'wing' to the other; that's the capsule. The inside of the capsule is lined with a thin, delicate substance called the synovial membrane. Normally the synovium's job is to nourish and lubricate the joint. In rheumatoid arthritis, the synovium is flooded by cells from your immune system, leading to thickening, what we call pannus. Although researchers have yet to discover why inflammation cells migrate into the lining of our joints, and why this inflammation is so persistent, we know that over time, the pannus can permanently damage the joint. Fortunately, although we can't cure rheumatoid arthritis, we now have medications that can control inflammation and prevent damage."

Lynn grimaced as she reached for my drawing and struggled to open the clasp on her purse to place it inside. As she reached forward, I noted a dark shadow of perspiration beneath each underarm. Then I pulled out my prescription pad. This was my second mistake. "In the meantime, I want to prescribe a low dose of a medication called prednisone. Short-term, it should quiet down the pain and swelling so that you can function better. It's not meant to be a long-term treatment, but a bridge between today and when slower-acting medications can control the inflammation. But first, let me tell you about possible side effects of prednisone..."

Her eyes flashed in terror. "Prednisone? Isn't that a steroid?"

"Yes...," and without skipping a beat, I reviewed the potential side effects of prednisone, how it was safe to take in small amounts in breastfeeding mothers, and works quickly to reduce pain and swelling, but that taking the drug long-term can lead to side effects such as weight gain, elevated blood sugars, and even brittle bones. A faint voice inside me was pleading, *go slower, be patient*, but I ignored it. "At the low dose I'm recommending, it's the most effective medication we have to quiet down severe arthritis inflammation."

"And do I have severe inflammation?"

"I'm afraid so."

She exhaled. "And, my baby? I'm breastfeeding. You can't, I mean, it's going to poison him too?"

A heavy silence hung over the room. After the miracle of childbirth, a doctor she barely knows wants her to take a medication that goes against every maternal instinct, every fiber of her being, but "poison?" I flipped through the patient information sheet until I came to *Diet: Vegetarian*.

Normally, I bond well with my vegetarian patients. I wish all of my patients were vegetarians. Dozens of studies have demonstrated that the *risk* of developing various diseases such as hypertension, diabetes, heart disease, even rheumatoid arthritis is reduced in vegetarians. But if diet was an effective treatment for serious immune system disorders such as RA, why do I regularly see patients like Lynn P. whose rheumatoid arthritis *began* while on a vegetarian diet? This is a difficult truth for some patients to accept: Diet matters, but is not a panacea. Sometimes horrific disease happens to good people on healthy diets.

I asked Lynn if she had been a vegetarian very long.

"I've been a vegetarian for ten years. No change there. Well…that's not exactly true," she added. "For the last two months, after this hit me out of the blue, I eliminated gluten and switched to a vegan diet. And last month, after reading about vegetables in the nightshade family triggering arthritis, you know, tomatoes, potatoes, sweet peppers, I took them out of the mix as well. To reduce the inflammation, I've been taking bromelain, borage oil, devil's paw, willow bark, fish oil, and turmeric." Her son stirred. Cooing in a soft, caressing, singsong lilt, she grimaced as she leaned forward and rocked the carrier until he settled down again.

"And has that helped?"

"They say it takes time for the toxins to be eliminated."

"The supplements may help with joint pain, to some degree, and by all means continue them, but in my experience, they don't improve this degree of inflammation." As soon as the words were out of my mouth, I could see her visibly stiffen.

"Why do you think this isn't Lyme disease?" Her voice was sharper, more confrontational.

I tried to reset my tone, hoping to make a therapeutic connection. "We see a lot of Lyme arthritis here in southern Maine. Most cases present with solitary swelling in a large joint, like the knee. What's more, patients with Lyme arthritis don't develop nodules at their elbows like you have. Your doctor tested you twice for Lyme disease and the tests have been negative."

"Can you test me again?" Lynn persisted. "I've read that the Lyme infection can hide and the test can be negative one time and positive the next."

"Of course," I replied evenly. I'll retest you for Lyme disease and add a test to rule out a viral trigger for your arthritis. In the meantime, would you consider taking a small dose of prednisone? You can barely function. It must be difficult taking care of your baby. Before starting the prednisone, you can ask your family doctor if they're comfortable with you taking a small dose while breastfeeding. At our follow-up visit, we can talk about other slower acting medications that can gradually take the place of prednisone. With some of the newer, slower acting medications, we can prevent damage and quiet down the inflammation so that you can function normally."

Quietly handing me back the prescription, Lynn agreed to the additional blood draws but not the prednisone. Then, cradling the baby carrier at the crook of her elbow, she limped ever so slightly down to the lab.

Returning to my office, I opened the chart of my next patient, lobsterman Ben Shipman, whom I had met nearly a decade ago while practicing on the Casco Bay Islands. Ben was not surprised when I diagnosed him with rheumatoid arthritis; his father and paternal aunt had both developed the disease in their early thirties and were "crippled" by their late 40s.

I referred Ben to Rheumatology Associates in Portland for management of his rheumatoid arthritis but continued to see his family at the clinic on Chebeague Island. Later that fall, after I'd missed the ferry, he offered me a ride in his lobster boat, HIGH MAINTENANCE, and showed me his hands. "I'm a good 70% better, maybe more, on the weekly methotrexate your rheumatology friends prescribed for me." As I observed Ben navigate his boat through a field of lobster buoys, it was clear that his wrists were still swollen, but by taping foam tubing around the wheel, Ben had a larger, more forgiving surface to wrap his fingers around. Marine radio controls had been changed out to larger, oversized knobs. He'd hired a sternman to help with hauling his 500 traps.

Five years later, when I joined Rheumatology Associates, Ben switched his care back to me. His disease had been slowed with what rheumatologist's call "disease-modifying drugs," but he was nowhere near remission. With each passing year his dexterity and grip strength were slowly declining. What's more, X-rays showed new damage to several of his knuckles, one knee, and the right wrist. We both knew he was failing.

Fortunately, in the year 1998, our office was participating in a clinical trial of infliximab (brand name: Remicade), one of the first "biologic" medications developed to block the activity of tumor necrosis factor (TNF), a key protein messenger in rheumatoid arthritis inflammation. Despite the time and distance of traveling to Portland from Chebeague Island, Ben readily agreed to participate in the study.

Today was his second clinic visit since starting the study and already, his joint inflammation was significantly improved.

Although there was an increased risk of infection with the use of Remicade, as one of my former partners commented to his patients, "There's nothing that I can give you as a medication that's worse than your disease."

The development of Remicade (and a host of new biologic medications in recent years) has radically altered the outlook for RA patients. Prior to biologic treatment, our goals of treatment: no pain, no joint damage, full function, were rarely met. Now, for the first time since he had developed RA, Ben's disease activity was zero.

At the conclusion of the visit, I asked Ben if he had any questions. "What about prevention?" he asked. "I've got two boys and I go to bed every night wondering when they're going to come down with it."

"First, I can't recommend strongly enough that the boys never take up smoking. In families with several members with RA, smoking is a huge risk factor for developing the disease. And diet? A vegetarian diet also lowers the risk of RA. There's a tremendous amount of research in this area, and I expect that someday, we'll have the tools to prevent RA in high-risk families like yours. Unfortunately, we're not there yet. I'm sorry."

That evening, as I cruised across the bay to Peaks Island in SAKAMO, I kept a sharp eye out for lobster buoys and floating debris in the half-darkness. Flocks of eiders and long-tailed ducks flushed off my bow, the skittish long-taileds first, the eiders nearly bumping into my bow before flying a short distance and resettling on the water. I slowed to headway speed to watch a seal slide off an ice flow into the water.

Could I have handled Lynn P.'s diagnosis and prednisone prescription more delicately? Yes. Knowing that she was breast feeding, I should have delayed treatment until she'd had time to come to grips with the diagnosis of rheumatoid arthritis. What if I'd sidestepped the issue of supplements, or at least put off the discussion until her second visit? After all, the supplements were not harmful and challenging their use only increased her distrust.

Off to port, a lobster boat caught my attention. I wondered if it was Ben Shipman, returning home to Chebeague Island. Patients like Ben knew firsthand how devastating RA could be to both an individual and their family and were more likely to accept aggressive medication treatment. I realized that my own reaction to Lynn P.'s skepticism about the diagnosis of RA and her insistence on sticking with natural treatments was also a product of my own family's trauma. My grandfather, Rice Beavers, a once vibrant blacksmith and West Virginia farmer, was crippled for the last seven years of his life from both Parkinson's disease and rheumatoid arthritis at a time when most patients failed to improve with standard care.

As I approached Peaks Island, my mind drifted to the emerging philosophy of shared decision-making in patient care. Here again, I had come up short with Lynn P. Patients deserve a voice in decision-making, to choose therapies consistent with their past experiences and worldview. As Brad Stuart, MD, and others have found in their research on healing, healing does not occur if patients are shamed for seeking alternate therapies, or if they're overwhelmed with data they cannot possibly absorb. To heal, patients must feel safe in being honest, making mistakes, asking questions—and in being guided, gently, by clinicians who care. This rebalancing of the physician/patient relationship, I agreed, was a healthy development.

But what if a patient chooses unwisely? What if Lynn P.'s fear of conventional treatment leads her down a path of lifelong pain and disability? Patients with RA don't get a second chance.

Once joint damage occurs it can't be reversed. Should an oncologist honor and accept the decision of a patient with a treatable leukemia to forego chemotherapy for supplements?

Tying up my boat to a finger pier, I ascended the ladder to the Peaks Island wharf and, opening up my pocket calendar, wrote: *Give Lynn P. a call next week*. Perhaps a brief chat on the phone after hours may help demonstrate my concern. Beneath the streetlight at the top of the hill, I noted that dressing in the dark 12 hours before, I had slipped on two different styles of shoes, one black, the other a rust brown. Perhaps Lynn P. had noticed. How much trust can you place in your doctor if he can't pick out a matching pair of shoes to wear each morning? More likely, I thought, the shoes weren't the problem. I was.

Chapter 10

From Peaks Island, the summit of snowcapped Mount Washington was partially obscured by clouds 70 miles to the west. The bay was flat, the sunrise softening the shadows extending out to House Island. Brad and I, his son Wyatt and my daughter Kate, both high school freshmen, boarded the Island Holiday ferry, lugging backpacks and skis, snowboards and boots, incongruous gear for mid-April even in Maine.

Several hours later, we arrived in the parking lot at the base of Mount Washington and gazed upward toward Tuckerman Ravine, a favorite destination for spring skiers and snowboarders. Then we shouldered our backpacks for the long ascent. Mud and clumps of fresh grass and mayflowers and wind anemone rimmed the trail as we trudged slowly upward. Spring flowers soon gave way to patches of snow, then deep drifts and frozen streams. When we arrived at the plateau at the base of the ravine, it was midwinter. A stiff breeze blew over the summit of Mount Washington, sending tendrils of snow down the headwall. I glanced at the thermometer dangling from my pack: It was 14 degrees.

As the least experienced skier (probably on the entire mountain), I was content to clamber my way partway up the headwall and snowplow warily down. The others, well, they went higher up the mountain, much higher. A small avalanche off to the left caught my eye as it swooshed down through an off-limits chute. Well above me, a skier caught an edge, teetered forward, and tumbled several hundred feet down the slope, Raggedy Ann limp, before she rose and bowed majestically to her friends at the summit.

By mid-afternoon, I was profoundly relieved when my daughter Kate announced that she was exhausted and asked if we could head down. Her eyebrows were caked in ice, her voice a croaky whisper. We chose a different trail to descend on the west side of the mountain along a stream pouring out of a snowfield. The trail was well trodden, other skiers were nearby, but an old saw of mountaineering came to mind: Most accidents happen going down the mountain. Kate was chattering away with Brad's son when, out of concern, I skied ahead and cut in between her and the stream. Then I abruptly lost my footing and slid over the bank and into the water, my backpack still attached, and was swept downstream.

Brad, who was slightly ahead of our group, dropped his pack and ran along the embankment. I floated over a ledge, collided with a boulder, spun into another boulder, and then, in the frothing shallow current, came to a stop. I was on my side, my upper torso barely above the waterline. I glanced downstream. Beyond the ledge where I was perched, there was no downstream. A roof of ice, thick enough to walk across, bridged the stream for as far as I could see.

From the bank, Brad shouted my name. He had taken off his belt and was in the water, calf-deep, straining to keep his balance. He stumbled and caught himself, the water threatening to sweep him off his feet.

I could feel the pressure of the current against my hand as I felt for the bottom, aware that any shift in my position might send me over the ledge and beneath the ice. I tried to reach out with my right arm, but it didn't seem to move normally. A wave washed over me, and I briefly shut my eyes. That's strange, I thought, I don't feel cold.

"Chuck! Grab the end of my belt!" Brad's voice seemed far away. I reached up awkwardly. There it was again, a deep, gnawing pain in my right shoulder. With my good hand, I closed my fist around the end of the belt, shifted my weight, and found bottom. The cascading stream was less than two feet deep.

Brad braced against an overhanging tree limb. "Don't look downstream!" I pushed away from the boulder, and balancing in the surging water, realized I was only a few steps from the bank. "Look at me!" Brad shouted. I raised my head. "Angle upstream. Small steps. Take your time." He pulled me in to shore. "There's a hut up the trail," he said over the din of the roaring creek. "It's not far. Can you walk?"

With my good arm wrapped around Brad's shoulder, I walked stiff-legged up the bank to the snow-packed trail. Several hikers arrived and wanted to carry me before recognizing that my shoulder was badly dislocated. "How far is it?" Brad asked.

"Maybe 200 yards," a woman answered. "I'll run ahead and notify the hut crew. They must have a first-aid kit and can radio for a snowcat." She looked at me skeptically. "Can you make it that far?"

"Shit, yes."

Brad peppered me with questions as he removed his wool cap and snugged it over my ears. "Did you hit your head? How old are you? Can you feel your hands and feet?" I looked at him dumbly. My mind seemed to be processing his words in slow motion. *Can you feel your hands and feet?* I slowly looked at my hands and feet and noted that my pants were icing up. I concentrated on moving forward. A few minutes later, inside the log hut, the crew stripped me down and sat me in front of a wood stove. I looked groggily at my shoulder. The upper part of my arm was displaced a third of the way across my chest. I was barefoot. Did I lose my boots in the water? Or did they take them off when they pulled my clothes off? I withdrew into my suffering. I'm not sure if I lost consciousness.

A snowcat arrived. Brad helped me to my feet and the crew, after wrapping me in blankets, laid me down. I couldn't stop shivering. I noticed that my arm was in a sling. On my uninjured side, Kate laid her head against my shoulder. She'd been crying, and I willed myself a smile. "I'm fine. I'm going to be fine," which I absolutely believed.

But I wasn't fine.

After a bumpy snowcat ride down the mountain, and a 30-minute ambulance ride to the North Conway Hospital ER where the emergency room physician reduced my dislocated shoulder, the pain dramatically improved. Following a hot sandwich and a liter of IV fluids, I wanted to go home. The ER doc saw no reason to keep me overnight. Kate, herself traumatized, sat in silence in the back seat of Brad's car with me for the two-hour drive back to Portland. "Once they popped my shoulder back in, my shoulder feels great," I lied to her. "I loved watching you ski."

We barely made the last ferry to Peaks Island that night. Back home, I retied my shoulder sling, swallowed several pain pills, and spent the first of many fitful nights, in and out of bed, taking hot showers to relax.

The nightmares began several nights later.

In my dreams I dropped repeatedly over the ledge and disappeared under the ice. I screamed and pounded against the undersurface in vain, attempting to break free. In some of my nightmares, I could hear the frantic voices of my daughter and Brad close by.

I developed a fear of darkness and closed-in spaces. Racing thoughts and flashbacks occurred when I least expected them, but most often in the half-darkness when I would awaken at night. In our bedroom, we kept a night-light on. We still keep a night-light on. I kept an anti-anxiety medication on hand. Sometimes I would take it. More times than I can count, deep within a nightmare, I would become aware of Sandi shouting, trying to pull me back from my terror. Night after night she watched over me, gently repeating the same message as she remained out of reach of my flailing arms. "Honey, you're okay. You're in bed. Wake up. Wake up."

Thankfully, and somewhat surprisingly, in between the panic attacks I seemed okay. I didn't suffer from chronic anxiety and continued my full-time medical practice. My ability to concentrate, to process information and formulate a diagnosis and plan, seemed unimpaired. I never saw a counselor.

A year later, somewhat better, I signed up for a leadership retreat in rural Maine. I did well during the day, but the first night without Sandi, when the lights went off in my cabin and I couldn't see my hand in front of my face, I jumped out of bed like a rabid animal and stumbled outside. Never mind that it was pouring rain and there was no porch. I spent the night huddled under a tree in my rain gear, awaiting first light.

Several years later, on a public health trip to South Sudan, I plugged my night-light into the wall of my room in a windowless, ramshackle rooming house. I was fine until midnight, when the power failed in the village and my room went dark. As I felt a rising panic, I slowed my breathing, willed my shoulders to relax, and kept my eyes tightly shut. Then, my panic bubbling to the surface, I leaped out of bed, crashed blindly down the hallway, and slept the rest of the night stretched out on a picnic table where I was feasted upon by mosquitoes. Several weeks later, back in the United States, I spiked a fever. After several courses of antimalarial medications, I recovered.

At some point, I forced myself to revisit the site of my accident on Mount Washington. At the edge of the stream, I sat quietly in the snow and felt the water's glassy power and beauty. There was no malevolence in the stream, I decided, only the relentless pull of gravity. Even so, I never looked directly at the roof of ice I would have disappeared under if I'd plunged over that last drop. The pilgrimage seemed to help. Last fall, for the first time in fifteen years, I spent the night alone in a tent. At one point I awakened and could barely see my hand, but behind it, through the mosquito netting, I could make out the stars. I relaxed and was able to go back to sleep.

Despite my gradual recovery, it would be misleading to say that I "got over" my trauma. A scar from a serious wound doesn't fade and disappear. The tissue heals, but the scar is fragile, more susceptible to re-injury. Facing my fears helped, but the accident remains with me, just beneath the surface. I'm fortunate that by and large, I've adjusted to a new landscape, a new me.

There are benefits. Putting on my physician's hat, I now realize that before my accident, I didn't truly understand the challenges my patients' faced with chronic anxiety, depression, or panic attacks. Sure, I tried to listen and identify emotional problems—particularly if they were a barrier to effective medical management. I ticked off the usual bromides: exercise, counseling, and medications, but inwardly, I was frustrated by my patient's inability to Just. Get. Better. Now that I myself suffer from a mental illness—post traumatic stress disorder (PTSD)— I think I understand. We all have something. None of us gets through this life unscathed.

Today, I hope I'm perceived by my patients as more empathetic, more accepting, perhaps kinder than I was before the accident. I know what it feels like to experience frightening symptoms and lose control. In recent years, I've worked out a truce with darkness and tight spaces. But I have my limitations. Just don't invite me to go caving and navigate through a black, constricting tunnel.

Years later, I'm down on a beach on Peaks Island with my 5-year-old grandson, Frank, Kate's son. It's dusk, and time to go inside. From a rusty culvert, water spills onto the beach and rushes seaward. Frank lugs sand and rocks to stem the flow but the water ultimately breaks through, submerging a toy dump truck and two Minecraft villagers. He stops for a moment and asks, "What's more powerful, wind, water, or an earthquake?" Then he answers his own question: "It's water."

I don't reply immediately. My eyes follow the stream as it twists and turns, tumbling sticks and leaves and bits of seaweed towards the surf. For a moment, as light is squeezed out of the horizon, I feel a cold chill. "Darkness too," I add. "Water and darkness. That's what I think. Did I ever tell you that I'm afraid of the dark?"

Frank reached over and placed his hand over mine. "It's okay, I'm afraid of the dark too."

Chapter 11

"…extraordinary care will be enhanced when we provide extraordinary caring."
Len Calabrese, DO

When Lynn P. finally returned to the office, I noted that she'd canceled several follow-up visits. Her husband, a lanky, pony-tailed man with an upturned handlebar mustache, wore baby Jett in a front pack. As I settled into a chair and opened her chart, Lynn struggled to open an envelope on her lap. When she dropped the envelope, her husband reached down, and without a word, placed it back in her hand.

"Well, I hope you have some answers for me," Lynn winced as she scratched her forehead.

"I do," I answered. "The laboratory testing for parvovirus was negative. The same goes for the repeat Lyme testing; it's negative as well." I handed the results to Lynn, who briefly glanced at the results before passing them on to her husband. "This last test, I've circled it in red, is for CCP antibodies, a highly specific test for rheumatoid arthritis. I'm sorry to say, it's markedly positive."

"But it says here…" she said, opening the envelope and handing me a copy of an article she'd printed from an internet site:

The Truth about Lyme disease: What your doctor won't tell you. "It says here that it's not unusual for patients with chronic Lyme disease to repeatedly test negative. I have so many of the symptoms of Lyme disease. I could have been bitten by a tick and not known it. More than 50% of patients don't have the rash."

I cringed at the implication that a physician would purposefully hide the truth from a patient and felt the gulf between us abruptly widening. Without opening the article, I handed the article back to Lynn. If this ends the visit, so be it. "I've seen this article before, but unfortunately, the symptoms you're referring to are not specific for Lyme disease. Patients with inflammatory arthritis have similar symptoms no matter what the cause." I paused as the baby Jett stirred and Lynn's husband retrieved a bottle from his backpack. "I wish you *did* have Lyme disease. Lyme arthritis can be cured with antibiotics."

Her husband spoke for the first time. "I think Dr. Radis needs to know that you've already done a course of doxycycline for Lyme through Dr. Barnes, and didn't that other doctor you saw, the Lyme specialist, didn't she combine another medication with the doxy for an additional month? You stopped breastfeeding but that didn't work. Now you're popping Advil and Aleve and the supplements, done the elimination diet, the copper bracelets. At our last visit with the Lyme doctor, she recommended four weeks of an intravenous antibiotic."

An uncomfortable silence settled over the room. Her husband continued. "I don't know if Lynn told you, but her aunt has rheumatoid arthritis. She tried the drugs. They didn't help and she had every side effect in the book. What was she on, Lynn? Gold? Chronic steroids?" Lynn silently nodded. "Now she hobbles around with a cane and sits all day in a chair. Some days she needs help getting up to the bathroom."

Now this was news. In fact, as I re-examined Lynn, I saw an opening in our conversation, perhaps a way forward. Lynn wasn't acting illogically, she was frightened. Her aunt had been prescribed injections of gold and steroids at a time when most patients with RA did poorly. We were in a different era, with far more effective medications, but Lynn's only previous connection to RA was her disabled aunt. No wonder she was skeptical of my recommendations.

The fact that Lynn had been treated unsuccessfully for Lyme disease could be my opportunity to initiate conventional medical management. As I methodically palpated Lynn's joints, it was clear that the disease had spread. The knees were visibly swollen and the motion in her right elbow was restricted to the point where she could barely flex the arm to comb her hair. With the increased swelling in her fingers and wrists, she was probably having trouble even wiping herself after toileting. Our window of opportunity to prevent damage and progressive disability was closing fast.

Finishing my exam, I summarized my findings. "At your first visit, you had eight swollen joints. Today, there are seventeen. Seventeen. If we further delay treatment for rheumatoid arthritis and the cartilage is damaged, it can't be undone. Because you are otherwise healthy—and that's a testament to you being a nonsmoker and your healthy diet—the risk of taking what we call disease-modifying medications is low. Today's medications are much more effective than the gold injections your aunt was treated with. With the right mix of medications, we can achieve our goal of putting this disease to sleep."

"Doc, she can't hold the baby." I noticed for the first time that her husband's eyes were puffy and bloodshot. They were both suffering.

"Then, as a start, I would recommend that I inject the wrists and knees with cortisone." Surprisingly, Lynn P. silently nodded her consent. I poked my head out the exam door and caught Joanne's eye. "Can you help me with several injections?" As I prepped the skin for the injections, I reviewed the pros and cons of taking methotrexate, a cornerstone of modern RA treatment. "Of course," I added, "every medication can have side effects. While on the medication, you'll need to avoid pregnancy, and we'll monitor your liver blood tests and blood counts regularly to ensure the medication is safe." I ended on a positive note. "There's good news. In recent years, we've found that the vitamin folic acid improves the safety of methotrexate, a great discovery."

Lynn leaned forward and for the first time asked a question. "You mean to say that a plain old vitamin is actually good for my inflammation?"

"Yes, indirectly. Folic acid lowers the risk of side effects from methotrexate and increases the likelihood you can take it long-term. We have a large number of patients who have taken methotrexate successfully for more than twenty years without complications. If we don't reach our goal of putting your RA to sleep, there's a new class of medications called biologic response modifiers, which I'm confident will help."

As she filled the syringes with cortisone, Joanne said to Lynn, "I noticed in your chart that you're a grade-school teacher. Just count yourself lucky you never had my son. When he was eight years old, the little sneak pulled the seat out from behind his teacher and she fell on her butt and had to be taken to the emergency room. Said he saw it on a TV show. My husband, he's a COP, when he came home, he chased Bryan around the house like the Gingerbread Man but couldn't catch the little bugger. What a scene. Now my son is a COP. Go figure."

That did it. Lynn, her husband, and I burst out laughing. The tension and distrust of the visit seemed to melt away. After I anaesthetized the wrist, the cortisone disappeared into the joint with only a tinge of discomfort. "There, one down," I rolled my swivel seat to the other side of the exam table. "Ready for the other wrist?

After the injections, Lynn P. flexed and extended her wrists and knees and smiled quizzically at how they could feel so much better so quickly. "It's the anesthetic," I said. "That will wear off later today, but it gives you a window into how we want your joints to feel going forward. In several days, the cortisone should kick in and the knees and wrists should improve again."

Lynn reached for her son Jett and cradled him against her chest. "The methotrexate can sound scary," I continued, "but so is this disease." I handed Lynn P. a slip of paper. "This is the name of a woman I treat for rheumatoid arthritis who owns an organic farm. She was also hesitant to take conventional medications. When I saw her recently in the office, she was doing much better and offered that she'd be happy to share her experience with other hesitant patients. Would you like me to ask her to give you a call?"

"That would be fine," Lynn P. nodded. "Thank you," she added. I picked up her chart to leave but she had one last question. "Bee sting therapy? I've read that the venom in the sting helps reduce inflammation. Can I combine bee sting therapy with methotrexate?" Lynn asked.

Without missing a beat, I readily agreed to the bargain. Our belief systems might never converge, but we shared similar goals: No pain. No swollen joints. Normal function. If the bees can work with methotrexate, certainly I can work with the bees. Let the stinging begin.

Chapter 12

After Lynn P. spoke with my organic farmer patient and reluctantly agreed to begin weekly methotrexate, her joint swelling and stiffness steadily improved. Three months into taking methotrexate, she achieved a long-term remission and offered to reach out to other patients who were reluctant to take immune-system medications. In this way, she helped me bridge the gap between "natural" approaches and conventional treatment. Of course, she also attributed a significant amount of her improvement to regular courses of bee sting therapy. And I was good with that.

But even as I adopted strategies to improve my connection to patients like Lynn P., another challenge arose. Women with silicone breast implants were increasingly referred to my office to determine if they had developed an autoimmune disease. These consultations delved into the complex world of law, multimillion dollar settlements, and junk science, and threatened the very basis of the traditional doctor-patient relationship.

I grabbed a fresh cup of coffee and caught a glimpse of my next consultation through the half-open door. Mrs. M. wore a white sweater and a long flowing cream-colored dress and was speaking to someone hidden beyond the exam table. Just before I ducked into my office, I heard her ask Joanne where the bathroom was located and watched her scurry down the hallway.

I had a few minutes.

I cracked open the records. First, some background. It is 1998 and each month I consult on two or three women with silicone breast implants who may or may not have an autoimmune disease. Without exception, they are in diffuse, excruciating pain and are convinced that the implants are the reason.

Whitman and Connolly, a New Orleans personal injury law firm representing thousands of breast implant patients has referred Mrs. M. to me to assess whether she qualifies for the Silicone Breast Implant Settlement. I opened her records and turned to the last page, the Disease Compensation Schedule. A menu of immune system disorders was listed. At the conclusion of my consultation, my job is to confirm a diagnosis and check off a box. The award, say, for a thirty-five-year-old woman with silicone breast implants and systemic lupus erythematosus is, my finger lingered over the number: 1.9 million dollars.

How did we get here? And why were so many women sick after breast implants?

Plastic surgeons Thomas Cronin and Frank Gerow are generally credited with performing the first silicone breast augmentation in 1962. For several decades, women quietly underwent the procedure with little fanfare. The implants could shift or leak, breasts could pucker or contract, but these poor outcomes were uncommon enough that the procedure remained popular. Of course, no one actually knew how often complications occurred. Oversight for breast implants by the Food and Drug Administration was minimal due to a grandfathering clause in regulations.

It was not until the early 1980s, when Ralph Nader's Public Citizen Health Research Group alleged that breast implants increased the risk of breast cancer, that the Food and Drug Administration began to give silicone breast implants a closer look. This potential linkage between breast implants and breast cancer was not borne out by further research. (In recent years, however, a rare form of lymphoma has been documented in the scar tissue *adjacent* to breast implants.)

The landscape for litigation dramatically changed when Maria Stern brought suit against Dow Corning in 1984, claiming that her autoimmune disease was triggered by her silicone breast implants. The jury awarded her $211,000 in compensatory damages and $1.5 million in punitive damages. In 1990, millions of television viewers tuned in to watch Connie Chung on a segment of "Face to Face" interview five women who believed that their silicone breast implants had triggered muscle and joint pain, rashes, and debilitating fatigue. Chung's show kindled a wave of uncritical media scrutiny. The number of individual lawsuits against Dow Corning ballooned to 12,359.

Individual jury trials slogged through the courts, and in fact, some juries did not find Dow Corning liable. When they did, however, the awards were huge. The cumulative impact of litigation brought Dow Corning to its knees. A 4 billion dollar agreement, the largest class action settlement in U.S. history, temporarily resolved the lengthy battles over causation. Dow Corning (and other smaller manufacturers) agreed to pay claimants a set amount of compensation for a menu of autoimmune diseases. All a patient needed was to be diagnosed by a board-certified rheumatologist with an autoimmune disease listed in the settlement.

That is where I came in.

I scanned through Hayden M.'s records and flipped to the tab: Laboratory Studies. Over the years, both before and after her breast implants, the majority of it was routine, the type of blood work one might draw for a yearly physical. These results were reassuringly normal. The immunologic studies followed. Of the ANA blood tests reported, one was before Mrs. M.'s breast implants, and two subsequently. The most recent was borderline positive. This was boldly underlined in red marker with the law firm comment: "*SLE test positive*."

I circled the conclusion with my pen. *Hmm…that's an untrue statement*. Numerous studies have documented that a borderline positive ANA can be detected not only in the blood of patients with autoimmune diseases, but in some patients with infection, with certain medications, and, at times, in healthy adults. It is *not* diagnostic for lupus. What's more, the ANA was performed at a specialty lab in Louisiana I was unfamiliar with. That's strange, I thought. There are plenty of good reference labs in Maine. If you want to be picky, the Massachusetts General Hospital has an excellent reference lab. But to send a lab specimen to Louisiana?

I flipped back to the title page in the notebook: Whitman and Connolly, New Orleans, Louisiana. A fleeting image of a lawyer objecting to his opponent's tactics flashed to mind, *You're leading the witness*!!

I'd read enough. It was time to see the patient.

Mrs. M. was tired, so tired it was all she could do to get out of bed most mornings. She patted the hand of the woman seated next to her. "Mother is a godsend those days I have trouble just putting one foot in front of the other. Plus, she's another set of ears. Honestly Mother, I can't count the times I've completely forgotten everything the doctor has said. Brain fog, that's what it feels like; I'm in a complete brain fog."

I looked up from my notes. "Other than the fatigue, how are you feeling?"

Mrs. M. pulled her shoulders back and sighed. "Weak. I'm weak. The pain is everywhere."

"We're fortunate that I live next door," her mother added, "On her bad days, I come over and help with the children, get them dressed, fix their lunches, get them off to school. Tom, her husband, is away frequently on business trips. I don't think he realizes…"

"And all of these problems? They go back how long?" I asked, shifting my attention back to Mrs. M.

"About two years after the breast implants," Mrs. M. whispered, almost inaudibly. "The fatigue, the pain, it slowly crept over me, until now, look at me. Is it the lupus? Is that what I'm struggling with?"

Momentarily, I said nothing. I gathered my thoughts, removed my glasses and cleaned them with a tissue paper. The diagnosis of lupus is not based on a collection of symptoms. It requires objective physical signs and significant widespread lab abnormalities. What's the difference between a symptom and a sign? It depends on who's able to notice it. Doctors can see or hear signs: a swollen joint, a rash, a heart murmur. Patients experience symptoms: fatigue, pain, difficulty with concentration.

I asked Mrs. M. to sit on the exam table. Her mother reflexively moved to her side and held an arm. "I'll be okay mother. Give me a moment. I'll be okay." I flashed back to the image of Mrs. M. hurrying down the hall to the bathroom. It didn't seem possible that this was the same person struggling to arise from a chair. Let it go, I thought. Now is the time to gather information, not draw conclusions.

Lupus patients often have discrete patches of hair loss. Hayden's scalp was normal. There was no rash across her cheeks. The inside of her mouth was free of ulcerations. Her heart and lung examination was normal. The breast implants did not demonstrate skin retractions or nodules. Next, I tested various muscle groups for weakness. Mrs. M. gave a good effort and I recorded in my notes: *normal muscle strength*. Her mother (as if she could read my mind), cleared her throat to clarify my exam. "Now today, she looks pretty good. She's giving you her best effort, but I know tomorrow, she'll be in bed all day."

"Mother. I will not. That's simply not true."

"It is so. Dr. Radis, I need to tell you something. Some mornings, when Hayden is bedbound, she calls and I come over and, like I said earlier, I get the children fed, dressed, and off to school. What I didn't say, those are the mornings, I have to feed her!"

"Well, she's lucky to have you," I said, half-listening, as I finished up with my neurologic exam. "It must be a great help for you to pitch in with the cooking…"

"No Dr. Radis," her mother said sharply. My head spooled round. "I'm saying I have to come over some mornings and FEED HER!" With that, the mother dipped an imaginary spoon into a bowl, pushed it towards Hayden's mouth, squeezed her cheeks, and inserted a spoonful of pretend cereal. Then she took out her handkerchief and dabbed her daughter's mouth. My reflex hammer fell to the floor. I sat down and recorded my findings, hoping to avoid eye contact with Hayden and her mother. "Some mornings, she's so weak," her mother continued, "I have to puree the food. That's a fact. That's what this…this boob job did to her."

"Okay. I think I understand," I sucked on the inside of my cheeks. There was not enough air in the room for the three of us.

My mind was on the verge of imploding, not to make sense of what I have just witnessed, no, that's the easy part. There is no medical disease that can fluctuate from scurrying down the hallway to the bathroom one day and needing help to chew the next.

I am absolutely certain that Mrs. M. and her mother will not be relieved to hear that she doesn't have lupus. The law firm of Whitman and Connolly will not be happy she doesn't have lupus. And frankly, I wish Mrs. M. did have lupus. There's treatment for lupus. With the proper medications, nearly all of my lupus patients are living well with their disease.

Joanne knocked on the door. "Dr. Radis, you have a phone call. If you have a minute, one of the cardiologists wants to discuss a hospital consult with you." I excused myself and gratefully took the call. My conversation with the cardiologist was brief, but allowed me to reset and refocus. After all, just because this was a breast implant consult with more than a million dollars riding on my evaluation should not, would not, alter my approach to Mrs. M. As a physician, my job is to listen, examine, diagnose, and treat. I am not a vending machine for the diagnosis of the week.

On my way down the hallway, I mulled over how I would explain to Mrs. M. that she didn't qualify for the Silicone Breast Implant Settlement, and wondered, could her symptoms represent Munchhausen syndrome, a disorder in which patients develop symptoms of a disease to gain attention? No, this didn't ring true. As a physician who has listened to thousands of histories, she seemed to genuinely believe that her fatigue and muscle pain were due to lupus.

I shifted my focus to Mrs. M.'s mother. Munchausen by proxy, the elaborate scheme by another (usually a mother) to transfer symptoms of a disease to a susceptible child, was another possibility. That Mrs. M.'s mother might be fueling her decline in order to share in a huge settlement was both unsettling and unprovable. As a non-psychiatrist I was in uncharted territory. Nevertheless, Mrs. M. deserved to know where I stood.

Inside the exam room, Mrs. M. sat to my right, her mother at her elbow. "Thank you for coming in today," I began. "This is a very complicated case. I need time to review the notes from the other consultants as well as the extensive lab your lawyer forwarded," I paused. Okay, so far so good. I turned my chair slightly towards Mrs. M. "Early next week, I'll get a letter out to your lawyer. I'll be calling your primary care doctor and reviewing my thoughts on how you can begin to feel better. For now, I want you to continue on the same medications you've been on…."

"Doctor," Mrs. M.'s mother interrupted me. "Now exactly WHAT is the problem? I am sick and tired of doctors putting her down. Are you going to sign off on the settlement or not? My daughter has lupus. She has that ANA and everything else. She's sick, sicker than you can imagine."

For a moment, I sat expressionless. I'd only have to open the settlement, check off the box for lupus, and I'd be done. Instead, I paused, exhaled, and said, "I'll go over your chart to see if I'm missing anything, and if I am, I'll be in touch with you. But from the information I have, no, you don't have lupus or another immune system disorder. I can't sign the settlement form."

Hayden stiffened, then began to sob. "I knew it. I knew it. You think I'm making all of this up. Well, it's real, and I hope someday you realize how wrong you are. I'm sick from the silicone. Sick." She brushed her hair back and dabbed her eyes with a tissue. "The silicone has spread everywhere in my body. Everywhere."

I never saw Hayden M. again, but her mother sent a letter threatening to report me to the Maine Board of Medicine. She never did. I don't know if the Louisiana law firm who sent her to my office sought a second or third opinion, but it was common knowledge at the time that certain rheumatologists were convinced that silicone breast implants triggered lupus and other autoimmune diseases and interpreted the evidence more favorably. Perhaps she was eventually reimbursed for her suffering.

The consult sat uneasily with me. At its core, the issue was not whether some women with breast implants had lupus or another autoimmune disease but whether this was happening more commonly than one would expect by chance alone. And the answer to this key question took time to answer. The health histories of residents of Olmstead County, Minnesota (where the Mayo Clinic is located) provided some answers. Public health researchers compared the health histories of silicone breast implant patients in Olmstead County with the women who did not undergo the procedure. The results, published in the New England Journal of Medicine, found no increased risk for developing lupus or any other autoimmune disease in silicone breast implant patients.

The next year, the Framingham Study, reporting on the long-term health of 87,501 women, also failed to demonstrate an increased risk for autoimmune disease in women with silicone breast implants. In all, 20 subsequent studies failed to demonstrate risk, while only two, one of which was published recently in 2022, suggested an increased risk. (The latest study was criticized by researchers because it was based on a review of medical records and didn't require confirmation of the diagnosis by an independent physician).

Eventually, I stopped seeing breast implant consultations; the office visits were uniformly adversarial. The women in the class action suit were not patients, they were plaintiffs. And while I sympathized with their pain and uncertainty, none of the thirty or so women I saw had evidence for an autoimmune disorder. Without exception, they were angry—angry at their surgeons who failed to warn them of potential complications, angry with Dow Corning and the FDA for marketing an unsafe product, and angry with me because I did not diagnose them with an autoimmune disease.

Juries and courts began to catch up with the science. In 1993, the U.S. Supreme Court established guidelines for determining what types of scientific evidence were allowed in court cases. The ruling made it more difficult for "junk science" to be presented to juries. It was the job of trial judges to ensure that expert opinions be based on reliable, reproducible science, not conjecture. Self-proclaimed "experts" were required to have credentials in matters they testified on. The Dow Corning settlement collapsed. Under a reorganization plan by Dow Corning to emerge from bankruptcy, women who wanted to cash out immediately and not file a disease claim were given $2,000, a far cry from the millions promised in the original settlement.

In the following years, I would occasionally see women who had signed up for the settlement but needed a local rheumatologist to manage their symptoms and gradually, I began to understand the powerful psychodynamics that prevented them from recovering. Over time, they transitioned from litigants to patients seeking advice. For the most part, my subset of silicone breast implant sufferers remained unwell. Several improved—to some degree—by having the silicone breast implants removed; others did not. I neither encouraged nor discouraged them from taking this step; I just couldn't predict if it would help.

Diffuse pain, fatigue, and anger were their constant companions. There was minor improvement with trials of prescription medications, from muscle relaxants to anti-inflammatories to antidepressants, but in my experience, yoga, tai-chi, physical therapy, and aerobic exercise were more beneficial.

One woman, who I followed for the better part of four years, helped me understand the mystery of why some silicone breast implant sufferers were more disabled than my worst rheumatoid patients. The answer, I believe, lies in the medical and psychological histories of women before they underwent breast augmentation.

Milly T. just wanted to feel better. She had been evaluated by two previous rheumatologists and both agreed that her breast implants had not triggered a connective tissue disease. Instead, they diagnosed her with fibromyalgia syndrome, a painful condition associated with normal laboratory studies, fragmented sleep, and often accompanied by depression and anxiety. And for the most part she accepted the diagnosis. But near the conclusion of our initial visit, I noticed in her new patient questionnaire that her mother had died at age 34 and asked Milly T. what happened.

"Murdered," she said simply.

"And...you were, how old?"

"Twelve."

"And your sisters?"

"Seven, ten, and fourteen."

"Well, I'm sorry." I whispered, and lay my pen on the desk. I was hesitant to explore the tragedy—I barely knew her—but I finally asked, "Do you want to tell me what happened?"

"No, well, actually…yes." She looked down at her lap, exhaled and whispered, "She was killed at home. It was a robbery and he...he, he shot her in front of us."

I closed my eyes, the image of that devastating, searing moment filling my mind.

"The guy was arrested a few days later at an elementary school where he was the janitor. Can you imagine that? He kills someone in cold blood and goes back to work scrubbing floors. He's in jail for life. But I wish they'd electrocuted him. It was tough. One sister died of an overdose. The other two drink. I mean, they're definitely alcoholics. Me…I saw a therapist for a while and was hospitalized when I took an overdose of Valium, finished high school, married too young, got divorced." She stopped for a moment and shrugged, "I sound really whacked, don't I?"

"No, I'm not surprised that your life fell apart."

"Well, for a while it did. But the next guy, Stanley, that's who I'm married to now, he's a peach. I mean, he's got a big heart. Getting the boobs helped. He liked them, still likes them, and then, like out of the blue, I'm f...cked again. The silicone implants are killing me."

Milly's story was extreme, but researchers have documented a number of differences between women who are seeking breast augmentation (as opposed to women undergoing breast implants after breast cancer surgery), and the general population. In nearly every measure of psychological health, from low self-esteem, to the incidence of preexisting depression and anxiety, to adverse childhood events, as a group, breast augmentation patients score lower than women who forego the procedure. While some women report improved self-esteem and other measures of improved psychological health after breast surgery, imagine the emotional trauma to a woman who is told her breast implants have triggered an incurable autoimmune disease?

The vivid imagery of poisonous silicone particles traveling throughout the body means you can't undo the damage. Sleep becomes fragmented and restless. Stress goes through the roof. Free-floating anxiety settles in. Headaches, fatigue, and diffuse pain worsen.

This, I believe, was at the heart of the silicone breast implant epidemic. Certainly, there were (and are) physicians and many patients who believed, and continue to believe otherwise. A perfect storm of circumstances—a susceptible population of women, initial reports linking silicone implants to autoimmune disease, media hype, and litigation—lit the fuse of disabling fear and suffering. Eventually, research failed to prove the connection between breast implants and autoimmune disease.

Over time, and with the help of a therapist, Milly accepted the connection between her mother's murder and her widespread pain. I shared with her my own story of how I developed PTSD following my winter skiing accident in the White Mountains and how traumatic events can trigger a flood of disabling symptoms. I suggested that she swim at the local YWCA, and six months later, she proudly announced she routinely swam 30 laps every Monday, Wednesday, and Friday. Her husband joined her on a daily evening walk.

I wish I could say that her symptoms melted away. They didn't. But her pain did improve, and she gradually tapered her muscle relaxants and stronger pain medications. The last time I saw Milly, she told me that her husband Stanley was still a "good guy." She was signed up for a 5K walk for PTSD survivors, and wanted me to know that she was working on forgiving the man who shot her mother.

Chapter 13

"Such a condition can put anyone on the shelf.
I know, because I suffer from it myself."
Robert Pettit, 2021

My mystery patient, Albion MacVane, rode shotgun in my Jeep on our way to a medical school class at the University of New England where I teach second-year medical students. Well past middle age, with a spidery build and a shock of explosive gray hair splaying over his ears, Albion rolled down the window and settled his deformed elbow on the edge of the door. There was a lump on the elbow. Actually, it was bigger than a lump; it was the size of a golf ball. And over the back of the hand was another growth, hard as a piece of quartz. I stole a glance at his fingers. They looked knobby and inflexible, but I knew they never stopped moving.

It was a bright warm late-spring, "finest kind" of day, and as we drove along, Albion had a kind word for everyone. Everyone, that is, except for the owners of several abutting farms who were suing him. They had no case against him, he insisted, not an ounce of proof, that *his* sheep farm, nestled on the distant ridge, had fouled *their* groundwater. And Albion proceeded to take me on a journey through the complexities of groundwater hydrodynamics, soil science, and animal husbandry. The man was no dummy.

I asked him why, since his arthritis began more than fifteen years ago, he'd never sought the advice of a doctor. He replied that maybe if he'd had a wife, she'd have brought him in sooner; he'd heard that women did that sometimes. Aspirin, "I buy it by the jug at Walmart," plus two generous shots of whiskey before bed helped him manage the pain. That is, until a ram knocked him down and he cracked two ribs, fractured the left kneecap and dislocated his left shoulder. His arthritis flared so badly from the trauma that when I saw him in consultation at the hospital—the man couldn't walk, dress, or feed himself—he agreed that it was time to take his arthritis flares seriously.

With the assistance of six cortisone shots, Albion went back to raising sheep. When I asked him at a follow-up office visit if he'd mind joining me at the medical school as a mystery arthritis patient, he agreed right off, and as we turned into the visitors parking lot, I reminded him of the ground rules: "First, the introductions. Then the students will ask you a series of questions about your arthritis. Remember to think back to when your inflammation was severe and you could hardly walk or use your hands. There's only one rule," I laughed, "they can't ask you what type of arthritis you have."

"Ruin the game," Albion said. "I'm the mystery in the room."

"Exactly. When we're done with the questions, I want you to walk up and down the aisles so they can examine your elbows and hands. Then I'll go to the blackboard, and this is the fun part, the class votes on your diagnosis."

"What if I don't know the answers to their questions? I'm no doctor."

"That's where I'll step in. But I don't think the questions will be too tough. They're second-year medical students. They don't know much. I think you'll do just fine."

"Oh, I'm not worried." Albion hummed a song and kept beat by lightly banging his stony wrist against the dashboard.

Inside the amphitheater 115 medical students settled into their seats as I pulled down the screen and handed my slides to the volunteer handling the projector. Albion took a seat next to me facing the students on the makeshift stage. "Mr. MacVane has been kind enough to visit with us today," I began. At this, Albion rolled up his sleeves and pointed to his all-too-obvious alien growths. "Remember, our focus today is to improve your ability to diagnose various forms of arthritis, and the best way to learn is to see and ask questions." Every eye in the room focused on our guest. "Okay, let's get going."

Five hands shot up. *This, I thought, is going to be awesome. Such enthusiasm.* A young woman in the front row posed the first question: "Mr. MacVane, thanks so much for coming today. Just how long ago did your arthritis begin?"

"You mean my gout?" Thud. Albion's hand shot up to his mouth. I looked up at the clock and shook my head. Eight seconds of mystery. Eight seconds. A nasal, trumpety snort broke the silence, and the amphitheater erupted in laughter. Several students looked like they were about to fall out of their seats. The tension of sitting for endless hours of lectures was broken by the absolute perfect comic timing of Albion MacVane. And Albion embraced the moment. He roamed the aisles like a rock star, demonstrating to the students his tophi (from the Latin word for stone), the uric acid deposits he had accumulated through decades of neglect. There was nothing more for me to add.

There is a saying in medicine, that sometimes the diseases are easy, but the patients are hard. This is particularly true in gout, where the triggers for the disease are well known, the diagnosis straightforward, and treatment often brings relief within hours of an acute attack. What's more, perhaps more than any other form of arthritis, diet matters. The risk of painful gout flares can be reduced by following a low-purine diet.

For those who continue with attacks despite dietary changes, the long-term daily use of a medication to lower uric acid levels usually prevents flares of gout altogether. Taking care of gout is often a high point in my day. One of my former medical partners so much enjoyed the AHA! moment of placing a drop of fluid from an inflamed joint on a slide and peering through the microscope to see the brightly colored uric acid crystals, that he daydreamed that he would someday advertise as a goutologist.

Historically, gout represents excess: excess in spirits, in diet, in debauchery, in girth. No one has captured the suffering of a gout attack as vividly as Dr. Thomas Sydenham (himself a gout sufferer) in 1683.

The victim goes to bed and sleeps in good health. About 2 o'clock in the morning, he is awakened by a severe pain in the great toe ... This pain is like that of a dislocation, and yet the parts feel as if cold water were poured over them. The pain which at first moderate becomes more intense. Now it is a violent stretching and tearing of the ligaments–now it is a gnawing pain and now a pressure and tightening. So exquisite and lively meanwhile is the feeling of the part affected, that it cannot bear the weight of bedclothes nor the jar of a person walking in the room.

Hippocrates, often referred to as the father of medicine, spoke nothing (and perhaps knew nothing) of rheumatoid arthritis or systemic lupus erythematosus, but recognized gout as a distinct form of corrupted humor with well-known predilections.

Hippocrates on gout:
VI-28: Eunuchs do not take the gout, nor become bald
VI-29: A woman does not take the gout, unless her menses be stopped
VI-3: A youth does not get gout before sexual intercourse

As for Albion, he was neither a eunuch nor a post-menopausal woman. His gout attacks were tightly linked to his regular consumption of red meat and alcohol, with a twentieth century twist to his attacks; he took a daily fluid pill for hypertension which further increased his uric acid levels. Understanding the development of gout attacks is fairly straightforward. Uric acid is the end product of our body's breakdown of purines. Purines are vital for our survival, but the more we ingest, the more uric acid is produced.

As an analogy, when salt is added to a glass of water, it dissolves. Add more and more salt to the water, however, and at a certain concentration, additional salt no longer remains dissolved and forms deposits on the bottom of the glass. In a similar way, when concentrations of uric acid are exceeded in the blood, needlelike uric acid crystals are deposited in the soft tissues of a joint.

Eventually, sometimes after an injury, or after a meal loaded with purines—a few beers, a steak—the crystals are released into the joint and a gout attack is triggered. To clean up the mess, the dirty work falls to our white blood cells, which flow into a gouty joint and release a fire hose of chemicals to break up the crystals. It is this cleanup process that gout sufferers experience as an acute attack. Over time, the white blood cells vacate the crime scene. Until the next release of crystals.

Thankfully, and somewhat surprisingly, Albion became a poster patient for gout medication compliance. Between stopping his fluid pill and faithfully taking a daily dose of a medication to lower his uric acid level, his uric acid level dropped into the normal range. What's more, he eventually made an honest, though imperfect effort to improve his diet and limit his alcohol to one shot of whiskey at bedtime.

In my early years in primary care on the Casco Bay Islands, I did not relish my encounters with gouty patients. Some of my patients were detached from my recommendations regarding diet and medications. My approach with these patients alternated between stern father figure and concerned friend. Honestly, in some patients—particularly alcoholics—nothing worked.

Take my former Peaks Island patient, Mike C., who regularly visited the Peaks Island Health Center with flares of gout. One afternoon, as he struggled to pull off his boot, he groaned, "The cherries stopped working."

Me: "Who told you to take cherries for the gout?"

Mike (genuinely surprised): "Why, I thought it was you!"

Me: "I'm quite sure it wasn't me. Are you still taking the daily allopurinol I prescribed to lower your uric acid and prevent attacks?"

Mike: "No. Should I be?"

Me (resisting the urge to whack my forehead): "Yes. Everyday." I wrote out my advice on a sticky note and instructed Albion to tape it to his refrigerator.

Take ALLOPURINOL EVERY DAY. It lowers your uric acid!

On second thought, I crumpled up the paper and tossed it in the wastebasket; this advice didn't work before, why think that he would follow my instructions now? It was time for a different tack. "Mike, this is your fourth attack this year, and sixth attack in two years. We're going in the wrong direction. What can I do to help you avoid gout attacks?"

Mike: "I don't know," he shrugged. "You're the doctor."

So much for shared decision-making. Me (drumming my fingers): "Okay. Remember the colchicine I prescribed recently? It's derived from a plant, the autumn crocus, and has been used for thousands of years for gout inflammation. When an attack comes on…"

Mike: "Oh! Now I remember. I ran out of colchicine. That works fine if I take it early, but I can never find it when I need it."

Me (looking back at my notes): "I wrote you a prescription for colchicine only three months ago with a year of refills."

Mike: "Refills? I threw the container away when it was empty. I have a nephew who visits from time to time, and I don't like him rummaging around in my bathroom. You know how kids are. Love him to death but he's always getting into mischief." We both looked at his great toe. If it was a thermometer, it would be on the verge of exploding.

Me: "The treatment of gout is like following a recipe. To make delicious food, you need to follow a recipe. To put gout permanently to sleep, you need to follow a recipe. If you can follow my suggestions, I'm optimistic we can prevent future attacks." I wrote on a sheet of paper:

1. *Reduce your red meat intake and use of alcohol!*
2. *Take Allopurinol every day!*
3. ***Don't stop allopurinol** with an attack of gout!*

4. Cherries are healthy. They're fine to take with an attack, but ***also take two colchicine*** *at the onset of an attack and one more two hours later.*

5. ***Then STOP the colchicine!!***

6. Remember ***alcohol is not medicine!***

Mike carefully placed my note in the front pocket of his shirt and promised that this time he would do better. Then he asked if I had time to inject his great toe. Injecting the great toe is akin to removing a toenail with a pair of pliers, but clearly, an injection was the only reason he had dragged himself to the clinic. As I drew up a dose of cortisone into a syringe, Mike grabbed both armrests of his chair like he was lifting off into space, all the while whistling *Wild Irish Rose.* It was an unexpectedly beautiful rendition. When I was done, he placed his boot back on, and leaning heavily on a makeshift cane, limped home. That was Mike's last gout attack. Something finally clicked. Or perhaps, it was the cherries.

Gout is managed routinely and quite successfully by primary care and only the most refractory, complex patients are referred to rheumatology. One such unfortunate woman, 55-year-old Mrs. Salter, looked like she could fit into my back pocket. Between her kidney failure from childhood onset diabetes and the need for a high-dose fluid pill, her uric acid level (despite her vegan diet and abstinence from alcohol) was the highest our laboratory had ever recorded.

At both elbows, two pebble-sized uric acid deposits protruded. Not as dramatic as Albion MacVane's, I thought, but still sizable. Where she out-gouted Albion was in the back of her heel where she had cut out a wedge in her sneaker to accommodate another stony growth.

Mrs. Salter's boggy, warm wrists were tender, not with the fire of acute gout, but with the unremitting agony of smoldering, chronic gout. Both knees were warm and swollen as were two fingers and the right ankle. All gout.

On the patient questionnaire, she wrote *Allopurinol—Rash! Liver abnormalities! The rash broke down and got infected!* So that's why she's not on daily allopurinol, the preferred, uric acid lowering, long-term treatment for gout.

Without a word, I flipped to the next page of her records. "Okay," I began, "has anyone ever talked to you about another medication called Uloric? Even in people who've had a serious allergic reaction to allopurinol, most people can take Uloric without side effects."

I crossed my fingers.

Mrs. Salter slumped in her chair. "My doctor prescribed it last spring; same result as allopurinol. Rash. I mean not just a rash but fluid-filled bubbles on my arms and legs."

I reviewed my options. There were not a lot of options. Pain medications such as ibuprofen or naproxen were out; they would further damage her fragile kidneys and tip her over into dialysis. Prednisone can control gout inflammation, but it raises blood sugars and wreaks havoc with diabetic control.

In cases like this, I'm sometimes left with the least bad option. The old saw, the diseases are easy, the patients are hard, in this case, was flipped. In ancient times, Hippocrates' patients rarely lived long enough with diabetes or chronic kidney disease to develop gout. Now my world is awash in it.

I reviewed her medication list again. The poor woman needed Oxycodone to control her gout flares. Buying time, I asked her how well the Oxycodone worked.

She considered this. "Well, you know, the Oxy*condom* does protect me from pain."

I smothered a smile and thought, *don't let the pharmaceutical companies get ahold of that quote.* Then I asked if anyone had ever aspirated and injected her joints with steroids.

"Yes. That was heaven," she brightened. "Of course, it only helped for a few weeks. Do you have time for that today?"

"Absolutely. Can we pick out several of your most painful joints?" I asked.

She pointed to both knees, the right wrist, and right ankle. "Those are the worst of the lot. I think if they were injected, I could get on and off the toilet without my husband helping me." Joanne methodically drew up four syringes filled with anesthetic and four syringes with a milky corticosteroid while Mrs. Salter looked on stoically. When I was done with the injections, she shook her head in wonder. "You numbed me up! Look at me! I can walk without a cane!"

I was not about to celebrate. There must be something I could prescribe to lower this poor woman's uric acid levels. Then I recalled Krystexxa, a newly released intravenous gout medication. I checked the Physicians' Desk Reference to ensure that it could be given safely with her degree of kidney failure, and the answer was a cautious yes. Of course, safely is a relative term. Only last week, I was called to the infusion room to evaluate a patient who suddenly developed a transfusion reaction 30 minutes into their first infusion of Krystexxa which had been prescribed by one of my partners. Thankfully, this resolved with an injection of steroids and epinephrine, but still required a trip to the emergency room.

"Mrs. Salter, I'm aware of the terrible side effects you've experienced with previous gout medicines," I said, "but there's a new medication which breaks down gout deposits and lowers uric acid levels. It's called Krystexxa and it's given as an intravenous infusion."

She flexed her knees and cautiously stood. A broad grin spread across her face. "You're saying this intravenous kryptonite might get rid of these stony lumps on my hands and feet?"

Ever the optimist, I nodded, "Yes."

The IV infusions worked. Six months after starting the new medication, Mrs. Salter arrived at my office without her cane. What's more, now that she was healthier overall, she was now a candidate for a kidney transplant. "My younger sister, bless her heart, is donating me a kidney. Look!" She pulled up a pants leg and the gouty deposits were barely palpable. "Oh, and I almost forgot, I have a present for you." She pulled out a small gift-wrapped box and handed it to me. "Before I met you, one of the hand surgeons removed one of the gout stones from my finger."

I opened the box. What a lovely gift for a rheumatologist. We walked down to the laboratory where I examined the slide under the laboratory microscope. After adjusting the focus, I exchanged seats with Mrs. Salter, who gasped at the appearance of the brilliant blue and yellow needlelike crystals. "No wonder I was so miserable," she said simply. "How can anything so beautiful be so frighteningly painful? I'm okay now," she decided, "and once I get my kidney transplant, I'll be even better."

Her luck held. The kidney transplant went off without a hitch. The new kidney worked so well that six months later, her fluid pill was discontinued, and I was able to eliminate the IV infusions of Krystexxa. He uric acid remained in the normal range. It was a remarkable 21st century twist to an old disease.

Chapter 14

The OxyContin Magic Show

"The greatest enemy of knowledge is not ignorance; it is the illusion of knowledge."
Daniel J. Boorstin

It was the late 1990s. The continuing medical education (CME) lecture in Rockland, Maine was titled: *Taking Chronic Pain Seriously,* and was delivered by an anesthesiologist from my community hospital. As I settled into my seat in the crowded auditorium, I kicked off my shoes and opened the syllabus. This could be interesting. After all, nearly every patient I see with arthritis has some degree of chronic pain. Little did I realize that the lecture would radically change the prescribing habits of nearly every doctor in attendance, including me. The house lights dimmed and our speaker stood at the lectern in the soft glow of a reading light.

First, similar to a magic show, there was *The Setup.* As a lecturer myself, I understood that the initial goal of any talk is to "hook" the audience.

The carefully crafted message, sprinkled with medical references to maintain the trappings of a scientific lecture, outlined our shortcomings. In slide after slide, physicians in the audience were gently chastised for not taking the needs of our chronic pain patients seriously. They are your friends and neighbors, we were reminded, your golf buddies, your colleagues. The chronic pain patient is the construction worker struggling to get up each morning for work, the fibromyalgia patient who tosses and turns all night, your elderly neighbor across the street struggling to maintain her independence.

We were reminded that chronic pain increases the risk of depression, leads to frequent absence from work, high rates of unemployment, and alcohol abuse. It was a national disgrace that physicians were not doing a better job managing chronic pain. As physicians, the lecturer continued, we wouldn't dream of under-treating pain in patients suffering with metastatic cancer. Why, then, don't we offer the same options to our chronic pain patients? Physicians such as Russell Portenoy, MD, a well-known pain specialist at Memorial Sloan Kettering Cancer Center in New York, suggested that the medical establishment suffered from "opiophobia," and claimed that the risks of long term-narcotics were overblown.

Next, *The Pledge*.

Our lecturer leaned into the microphone and delivered the pitch: the solution for long-term management of chronic pain was with opioids, preferably with OxyContin, a twice daily sustained release drug with a favorable side effect profile. I flipped to the back page of the conference materials and noted the sponsor for the talk was Purdue Frederick Company, the makers of OxyContin. Never heard of them.

Despite my vague uneasiness that I was being manipulated, I found myself quietly agreeing with the basic premise: It's time to take the unmet needs of our patients with chronic pain seriously. But what about addiction? What about diversion? What about tolerance? Where is the data? The lecturer, seemingly able to read my mind, clicked to a series of small print slides to address my concerns. I leaned forward to read the data. I couldn't read the data. He summarized the data. Click, on to the next slide. Phrases such as *the risk of addiction is overblown* haunt me even today.

Finally, there was *The Close.*

Like a master magician, there had been misdirection—`drawing attention away from the primary goal: Sell More OxyContin! Next, a false perception was created, influencing behavior without doctors realizing they were being manipulated. The anesthesiologist concluded his lecture with a warning. There had been the carrot, now, the stick. Not only was it important to recognize and treat our patients' chronic pain, but not doing so risked sanctions from our state medical societies and perhaps, lawsuits.

According to Patrick Radden Keefe, the author of *Empire of Pain*—a scathing history of the Sackler family and their promotion of OxyContin through their family-owned business, Purdue Pharmaceutical L.P.—I was on the receiving end of a sophisticated infomercial aimed at changing my behavior. And it worked. Whether they admit it or not, nearly every physician who followed patients with chronic pain who sat through an OxyContin "educational" lecture was influenced by this campaign.

In the following months and years, Purdue instructed sales representatives to follow up with visits to physicians' offices, driving home a series of talking points. Purdue instructed sales representatives to assure doctors (repeatedly and without evidence), that fewer than one per cent of patients who took OxyContin became addicted. In fact, according to Patrick Keefe, the company's own records later revealed the incidence of addiction to OxyContin was much higher. In one study (commissioned by Purdue Frederick but never published), 29% of patients in West Virginia who were prescribed OxyContin for chronic headaches became addicted.

At the end of the presentation, I was an agnostic, not a true believer. I noted that our lecturer presented only a single study demonstrating that narcotics can improve chronic, nonmalignant pain. His review of the study was superficial, and the duration of the study was relatively short. If we were to change our paradigm for treating long-term chronic pain, didn't we need more data?

The stage had been meticulously set. A few years earlier, in 1995, the same year OxyContin was approved by the Food and Drug Administration (FDA), Dr. James Campbell addressed the American Pain Society and urged healthcare providers to add pain to the traditional four vital signs: blood pressure, respiratory rate, temperature, and heart rate. A 10-point pain scale was soon adopted by hospitals and physician practices throughout the country, instructing care providers to treat pain as the fifth vital sign.

The inclusion of pain alongside the traditional vital signs was not without controversy. Some physicians pushed back. Changes in vital signs may have serious implications: infection, heart attack, stroke. Pain, on the other hand, is a symptom, an individual experience. Pick a number and it is true, or as one of my medical partners once commented, "One person's 10 is another person's 3." Was treating acute or chronic pain really as simple as a patient reporting a number?

But even as an agnostic, even with the natural tendency for memory to gloss over past mistakes, I must admit that I was subtly co-opted by the lecture. Despite my misgivings, my behavior changed. Even an agnostic may attend church now and then.

Rheumatologists have always prescribed opioids for patients with chronic pain, but it was a small subset. For instance, patients with bone-against-bone arthritis in whom joint replacement surgery was too high of a risk often reported that low-dose narcotics allowed them to adopt healthy behaviors such as swimming or yoga to maintain function and reduce pain. Almost none of these patients became addicted.

What was different now, was that we were awash with patient requests for narcotics. Some of these patients, as they say in the business, "were not good candidates." They had severe, chronic back pain with minimal arthritis or suffered from untreated post-traumatic stress disorder (PTSD) or severe depression or chronic anxiety. We now know that these patients are at higher risk for opioid addiction.

One of the physicians in my practice was a narcotic Luddite. He rejected the notion that treating chronic pain with narcotics was an ethical imperative and believed that there was no convincing evidence that they were effective in treating chronic pain. If an arthritis patient requested OxyContin, he simply told them to take up their request with their primary care provider, or referred them to a pain specialist.

There were sophisticated ruses used by addicts.

My first experience was with a new patient to my practice. Smartly dressed in a button-down blue shirt with creased slacks and Top-Sider boat shoes, he claimed that he had recently moved to Maine from Pennsylvania for a new job. He brought no records but filled out his patient questionnaire in detail. An X-ray I obtained that morning demonstrated bony spurs throughout the lower spine (what is termed a "bamboo spine") and a fused sacroiliac joint. The diagnosis: ankylosing spondylitis, one of my diseases. The patient was in the right office.

Our conversation turned to previous medications he had taken. Ibuprofen had triggered a bleeding ulcer. Prednisone had led to uncontrolled blood sugars. When his doctor prescribed OxyContin for his back pain it had worked. It was the first time in years that he slept through the night.

The patient was grateful that I was seeing him; he was nearly out of his OxyContin prescription and hoped I could continue it. With it, he could go to work; without it, he was nearly bedbound.

I filled his prescription, perhaps raising an eyebrow at the unusually high dose he claimed to be on, and made an appointment to see him in follow-up in one month. A week later I was called during office hours by the police from a neighboring town. My patient had been found dead, slumped in a bathroom stall with a syringe dangling from his arm and an empty bottle of OxyContin and a cigarette lighter on the tile floor. He had melted down and injected the drug. My name was on the bottle. In his wallet were three photo IDs of him with three different names. Was there anything I could tell them about this man? It was embarrassing to admit, but I had met him only once. Yes, I had written the prescription. No, I didn't know he had recently been released from a halfway house in Pennsylvania.

I had been duped.

In another case, I consulted on a middle-aged woman who lived in a rural community several hours north of Portland. At least 30 pounds underweight, she was a sad, frail, wisp of a woman with extensive joint damage from rheumatoid arthritis. Her partner, who was twice her size, did much of the talking, often finishing her sentences and telling me repeatedly just how much pain she was suffering from. I found myself increasingly irritated by this. When he had finished yet another sentence for her, she looked down at the floor and quietly said, "Yes, I think that's how I feel."

After finishing my exam, I lightly touched her hand and said, "I believe with a change in your medications, we have a good chance of controlling the inflammation and reducing your pain."

"I'm all in favor of that," her partner brightened. "The OxyContin her doctor prescribed worked like a charm. He's moved on. He was only a temp. She was pain free when she was on the Oxy."

"From the sound of it," I said, acutely aware that her partner's single-minded focus on pain medications rather than the bigger picture of controlling her inflammation was a red flag. I spoke directly to the woman. "From the sound of it," I repeated, feeling my way along in an increasingly uncomfortable interaction, "it's been years since you've been prescribed what we call in rheumatology, a disease-modifying medication. Going forward, my goal is to reduce pain by controlling inflammation and improve function by working hand in hand with a physical and occupational therapist."

Her partner considered this. The woman continued to stare emotionlessly at the floor. "You mean to say, that in addition to the Oxy, she needs other medications? That's fine," he decided. "She's good at taking pills."

"No." I turned to meet his eyes. I was learning to trust my instincts in this new world of chronic pain management. "I mean that my focus will be on the treatment of her rheumatoid arthritis. Reducing inflammation will reduce pain. If we don't meet that goal, I may add a narcotic, not before."

"That don't make no sense," his voice had an edge to it. "She's done just fine on the Oxy. I hear those other medications have side effects." He crossed his arms. It felt like a threat.

I ignored him and turned back to my patient. After reviewing potential side effects of weekly methotrexate and the need for regular blood work to ensure its safety, I handed her the prescription. The visit was over. I didn't look back. Once out of the room, I leaned against the wall and closed my eyes to clear my mind for the next patient.

Over lunch, Joanne called the patient's local pharmacy to verify her other medications. After a pause, the pharmacist noted that the patient's OxyContin prescription had been filled only a week previously by another physician and was relieved we were not prescribing the drug. "As a matter of fact," he added, "I've had several calls about her in the past month. Apparently, she's obtaining OxyContin from a number of practitioners."

I suspect, but don't know with absolute certainty, that the unfortunate woman was being trafficked for drugs. I never saw the couple again. As the epidemic spread, patients who would normally be considered at low risk for addiction became victims of the increased accessibility of narcotics. High school football players became addicted after liberal prescriptions for narcotics following fractures. Mothers and fathers of school-aged children became hooked after prescriptions for back pain or headaches. Teenagers experimented with OxyContin at parties. Laborers, accountants, and small-business owners transitioned from prescription OxyContin (and other narcotics) to street drugs when their prescriptions were discontinued. No group was immune.

Purdue Pharma (owned by the Sackler family) has been sued for its role in promoting OxyContin. A number of these cases have been settled. No one from the Sackler family has gone to jail. In Maine, despite controls on narcotic prescriptions, the number of fatal drug overdoses remains unacceptably high. If the 1990s were the decade of prescription opioids, the next decade was dominated by heroin, and in recent years by fentanyl. The problem of patients going from doctor to doctor seeking narcotics would not be addressed until a statewide prescription monitoring program in Maine was established in 2003. Since then, patients can no longer fill narcotic prescriptions from multiple providers. But the damage had been done.

Today, some physicians never prescribe opioids for chronic pain, or if they assume the care of a patient whose doctor has moved or retired, the patient is required to taper down and discontinue their narcotic. This rigid black-and-white attitude has left many patients bewildered and angry. One of my former patients with severe destructive RA, who felt that low-dose narcotics had helped her cope with chronic pain, confided that she felt like a drug addict each time she refilled her narcotic prescription. The stigma is back.

In response, the New England Journal of Medicine in 2018 sought a middle ground. “As the pendulum swings from liberal opioid prescribing to a more rational, measured, and safer approach, we can strive to ensure that it doesn’t swing too far, leaving patients suffering as the result of injudicious policies.”

If narcotics are not the answer for most patients with chronic pain, what is? There is hope that cannabinoid derivatives may offer meaningful relief from chronic pain. A number of my patients with rheumatologic conditions are experimenting with cannabis products; some believe it helps, others do not. According to Dr. Fitzcharles at the Louise and Alan Edwards Pain Management Centre in Canada, “To date, there has been very limited study of pharmaceutical cannabinoid products in rheumatic diseases…and less convincing evidence for benefit. There are no published randomized clinical trials of herbal cannabis in rheumatic diseases.”

Doctors are trained to gather information, assess the data, and make evidence-based decisions. At a presentation I attended recently, the lecturer stated that cannabis was the answer to a host of medical conditions, including chronic pain. He blew through a series of slides, and summarized the data from several small studies in the same pseudoscientific manner the OxyContin lecturer did years before. The presentation ran through the allotted time slot. There was no time for questions. I quietly seethed in my seat.

I await the results of well-controlled, long-term studies in the diseases I treat before I become a true believer in the use of cannabis for chronic pain. In the meantime, a number of well-designed studies have shown that self-help measures such as stretching and light weight lifting, swimming, yoga, and tai chi programs, and cognitive behavioral therapy can lead to a reduction in pain and improved quality of life. For patients willing to do the work, these modalities are a welcome alternative to the chronic use of narcotics.

The OxyContin magic show was an illusion. Physicians and their patients believed in the magic message. And we're still paying the price.

Chapter 15

"Pain is inevitable. Suffering is optional."
Buddhist saying

Mrs. Frent removed her shoes and placed her handbag on the adjacent chair before she stepped gingerly onto the scale. Her weight recorded, she groaned as she picked up her handbag and slung it over her shoulder. I glanced in her direction. Pear figured, early 40s, she was moderately overweight with several varicose veins winding their way down one leg. The right hand looked normal. The left hand looked normal.

Joanne led her into exam room #5 as I reviewed her internist's notes. *Married, two children, ages 8 and 11, works full-time, one-half pack a day cigarette smoker.* The medical problem list was relatively short: *anxiety, irritable bowel syndrome, migraines, chronic insomnia.* In the margin of her most recent note her doctor had penned: *Severe fatigue, trouble concentrating... widespread muscle and joint pain. Lupus*?

Deeper into the chart were the results of various laboratory and imaging tests. I flipped through the results; for the most part, these were all uniformly normal. I paused at the report of an MRI of the lower spine: *mild degenerative disc disease changes.*

"The dreaded degenerative disc disease diagnosis," I commented to the internal medicine resident who was spending an afternoon with me in the office. "It's an unfortunate phrase. As we age, osteoarthritis is invariably seen on X-rays of the spine, even in people who have never had a day of back pain in their entire life. Why this has become a go-to phrase in a radiology report is a mystery to me. The phrase, *degenerative disc disease* triggers anxiety in some patients that can never be dispelled. One of my fellow rheumatologists once described these changes as normal abnormalities consistent with being human."

I closed the chart, opened the door, and greeted my new patient. "Good morning. Is it okay if another doctor joins us?"

"Of course. Of course," she waved us both in.

"So, when was the last time you were well?" I began.

She cocked her head, considering this. "Like, not in pain?"

"Yes." I waited.

"I can't remember not having pain. The pain is excruciating. My dad used to tell me that I was born with old parts. When I was a little girl, my mom would massage my legs at night. The doctor called it growing pains. Headaches took hold during my teenage years. Don't talk to me about my bowels. The gastroenterologist calls it irritable bowel syndrome, but it's miles beyond irritable. Between the diarrhea and constipation, some days I feel like I could pass out on the commode. Oh, I fell on the ice in college and that's when my back pain settled in. At night, I start on my back, but that's no good, so I roll on my side. Then my hips, they're on fire, so I lie on my stomach, but that puts a strain on my neck. All night long I'm turning like a rotisserie. I'm a mess!"

On her patient questionnaire, Mrs. Frent had colored in the skeletal figure where she had pain; only the central face was spared. I asked her the usual questions, whether she had frequent ulcers inside the mouth, hair loss, unusual rashes, or joint swelling. The answers were reassuringly normal. One thing for sure, the patient did not have lupus.

I stepped out of the room with the internal medicine resident while Mrs. Frent changed into a cloth gown. “So…any thoughts? Can you give me your differential diagnosis?”

“Well,” he offered, scratching the back of his head. “I mean, she could have lupus, couldn’t she?”

“Hmm… hold that thought. I think she’s changed by now.” I knocked softly on the door and reentered. Mrs. Frent reported considerable discomfort as I gently squeezed the wrists and individual fingers but there was no redness or swelling in the joints. She flinched, well, nearly everywhere I pressed firmly against the skin with my index finger.

When I palpated the outer hips and asked her to pick a number on a scale of one to ten, with ten being the worst pain she had ever experienced, she said, “EIGHT!” Then I pressed on the soft tissues adjacent to the lower spine and she groaned, “ELEVEN!” I’ve utilized this pressure/pain assessment on hundreds of patients, and her answer of ELEVEN! was noteworthy. It implied a level of suffering I don’t see in even my most crippled arthritis patients.

I switched to another topic. “Can you tell me more about your sleep?”

“I never sleep.” It seemed an odd answer. We all sleep. Sometimes our sleep is of poor quality, but never sleeping?

“Every morning, I’m more tired than when I went to bed. I feel beaten up, bruised, like the flu, only worse. When I try to go to sleep, my mind won’t turn off. It’s like an endless film clip.” I jotted down noteworthy stressors that could impact sleep: *primary caregiver for elderly mother-in-law, son with ADHD acting out, money worries, discord at work, husband doesn't understand her pain.*

After finishing my examination, I asked her to get dressed, and retired to my office with the internal medicine resident. "Okay, the diagnosis is…?" I asked, as I divided a fresh white sheet of paper into three columns.

"Fibromyalgia syndrome?" he answered, more confidently.

"Good, I agree. She fulfills the criteria for the diagnosis: widespread musculoskeletal pain and tenderness of greater than three months duration, fragmented sleep, and a lack of evidence for an alternative diagnosis such as an underactive thyroid, lupus or Lyme disease. Although the pain may be severe, even after many years, fibromyalgia pain doesn't lead to damage of the muscles or joints.

"Importantly, there are a multitude of stressors in her life, some of them very chronic and not easily resolved. But I want to emphasize, fibromyalgia is not merely a symptom of chronic anxiety or depression," I continued. "Not all anxiety or depressed patients have chronic pain. Not all fibromyalgia patients have chronic anxiety or depression. Having said that, the three conditions are frequently seen together.

"We have a few minutes." I took out a blank sheet of paper and divided patients into three subgroups.

<u>Fibromyalgia Syndrome:</u> <u>Patients with an excellent response to treatment.</u>

Pain and insomnia of recent onset. Current stressors may be high but are not unsolvable. There is good support from friends and family and a past history of regular exercise The patient is a non-smoker and not addicted to alcohol or drugs.

"This patient might be a young mother who played on her high school soccer team. She is working full-time, up frequently at night with two-year-old twins, and now has widespread muscle achiness and fatigue. She's worried that an underlying disease is triggering her pain. When a diagnosis of fibromyalgia is made, patients in this subset are often relieved. These patients want to avoid taking prescription medications, and despite their busy/stressful lives, they're interested in self-help measures such as exercise, yoga, or tai chi.

At their follow-up visit, the patient is usually improved. Her partner is splitting the nighttime bottle feedings and she is sleeping better. A friend comes over to her house several times a week and watches the twins while she goes for a 30-minute walk. On weekends, her partner takes the children to the playground while she attends a weekly yoga class. Her symptoms may continue to wax and wane but she embraces the mind-body connection as a contributor to her muscle and joint pain and the importance of regular exercise, stress management, and restful sleep."

Fibromyalgia Syndrome: Patients with a partial response to treatment.

Symptoms are chronic. There is often a current or past history of anxiety, panic attacks, and/or depression, and sleep problems are long standing. Stressors are present with little likelihood of resolution. Social support is fragile and sometimes unhelpful. Patients in this subgroup may feel they don't have time to exercise or may experience increased discomfort with exercise.

"As an example, let's go no farther than our new consult. Her problems with sleep have been present for years. In addition to working full-time, she is the primary caregiver for her mother in-law and has a son with behavioral problems. Work is unsatisfying." I pointed to a line she'd filled out in her patient questionnaire: *My husband doesn't understand my pain.* "Not much emotional support there."

"I often prescribe medications such as Cymbalta or Lyrica or Savella for this group of fibromyalgia patients, but to be honest, improvement is rarely life-changing and medications are often discontinued due to side effects. Patients may dabble with exercise but if they experience increased discomfort, they remain inactive. In my experience, cognitive behavioral therapy can improve quality of life in these patients, but it's challenging to convince patients that a therapist can help."

Fibromyalgia Syndrome: Patients with a poor response to treatment.

Symptoms are chronic and often debilitating. There is ongoing mental illness which may include adverse childhood experiences including sexual or physical abuse. Social support is poor or nonexistent. There is current heavy use of cigarettes, and/or alcohol or other drugs. The patient may be on opioids for chronic pain but pain continues to be severe. Patients in this subset are often unable or unwilling to exercise due to pain and have trouble agreeing to or accessing counseling.

"Working with these patients may be frustrating for both the patient and their healthcare providers, in part because their lives are often chaotic. It's particularly important in this group to avoid polypharmacy—prescribing multiple medications to manage mental health disorders, insomnia, and pain. Unfortunately, because of the intensity of their symptoms, it's this subgroup that is often prescribed narcotics for pain, which are ineffective or paradoxically may make their pain worse. Let's go back and talk with our new patient and I'll flesh out my approach. This isn't a condition you can manage by following a computer-generated list of recommendations."

Thirty minutes later, I felt more exhausted than after a difficult visit with my sickest autoimmune disease patient. At first, Mrs. Frent politely listened to my explanation that, thankfully, she did not have lupus—which she was convinced she had—but instead suffered from fibromyalgia syndrome. I was optimistic, I told her, that by working together, her pain and quality of life could be improved. Abruptly, I could feel the atmosphere of the visit shift as she processed what I had said.

"So, you mean to say that all this pain I'm suffering with is in my head? Is that what you're saying?"

"No, the pain is real." I slowed down, aware that I was about to lose her confidence. "It is as real as symptoms of headache or chronic fatigue or depression—all conditions with normal laboratory results and physical exams—but the science is pointing towards the central nervous system and the way it processes pain as the real culprit in fibromyalgia. How do we know? We can trigger fibromyalgia symptoms in healthy volunteers by withholding deep restorative sleep. That's what Dr. Harvey Moldofsky did in Canada some years ago."

I had her attention. She sat back down and loosened her grip on her shoulder bag.

"For the experiment, the volunteers reported to Dr. Moldofsky's sleep lab where technicians attached electrodes to their scalps."

Mrs. Frent leaned forward in her seat. "What was being measured?"

"Brain wave activity. You've probably read about levels of sleep and brain wave activity, right? Well, Dr. Moldofsky wanted to see what happened when he deprived his volunteers of stage IV delta wave sleep, the restorative kind of sleep that we wish we had more of."

"And what happened?"

"Now mind you, the technicians did not deprive the volunteers of all sleep, just stage IV sleep. After only a few days, the volunteers developed widespread pain."

"They developed fibromyalgia?"

"Yes, but some fared better than others. Those who exercised during the day despite their fatigue and fragmented sleep fared better than those who felt too tired to exercise. After the study ended, the volunteers gradually returned to their normal sleep cycles. When they were reexamined several weeks later, they no longer had widespread pain. What do you think that tells us?"

"So maybe I need a sleeping pill or pain pill to knock me out?"

Internally, I cringed. "You would think so, but unfortunately, it's not that simple. Sleeping pills don't seem to help the pain of fibromyalgia syndrome. But we do have medications for fibromyalgia. For instance, Lyrica is…"

"Oh, my goodness! I was in a fog when I took Lyrica."

Now this was news. Evidently, Mrs. Frent hadn't filled out her patient questionnaire completely prior to our visit. I recalibrated. "Have you taken anything that has helped?"

"No, not really. Motrin is like eating candy. Tylenol is worthless. The pain is head to toe, 24/7; it never sleeps

"Any other medications?" I asked.

"My doctor also prescribed a nighttime dose of a depression medication, but it turned me into a zombie. Same goes for the muscle relaxant. I don't know how I go on. I have a high pain threshold but the pain is excruciating."

I lifted an eyebrow. There it was again, the word excruciating. The word implies a level of suffering rarely associated with other disorders rheumatologists treat. One of my former partners offered this observation: "If a patient describes their pain as excruciating, fibromyalgia syndrome is the diagnosis. If they use the word twice in the same visit, their pain is untreatable." This remark may sound unkind, but research suggests that there is truth to the observation that how pain is processed and expressed plays an important role in how a patient lives with chronic pain.

Melanie Thernstrom, in her book, *The Pain Chronicles,* describes the tendency of some chronic pain patients to "catastrophize"—to embroider pain with fear and anxiety—resulting in enhanced central nervous system activity and more pain and anxiety. The vivid images Mrs. Frent used to describe her pain are almost never described by my patients with immune system disorders such as rheumatoid arthritis or lupus. This may create an empathy gap between the practitioner and the patient. We simply don't have medications which can manage the suffering induced by an icepick or an internal explosion.

The phrase, "I have a high pain threshold," is another comment often heard in patients with fibromyalgia. Unfortunately, the opposite is usually true. In studies using a dolorimeter, an instrument which applies consistent pressure to the skin, we know that patients with fibromyalgia syndrome experience discomfort with lower levels of pressure than patients without the disorder.

Current evidence suggests that fibromyalgia is not an autoimmune or inflammatory disorder. It is a pain threshold disorder, a complex amplification of pain pathways within the central nervous system in which normal everyday discomfort is experienced as pain. From previous consultations, I know that explaining fibromyalgia syndrome as a pain threshold disorder may not go over well. To the patient, the explanation may sound unconvincing, even demeaning. I wanted Mrs. Frent to leave my office today with the tools to manage and improve her pain.

"So, what *can* I do for the pain?" Mrs. Frent asked. "And don't say get out and exercise. I went out for a walk last week and afterwards, I was in bed for the better part of two days."

None of this boded well for her recovery. Exercise plays a critical role in managing chronic pain. Even so, I persisted. "If you're unable to walk, how about yoga, tai chi or a therapeutic swim class? A number of studies have shown that patients who regularly participate in one of these programs can reduce their pain long term."

"And how exactly am I going to find the time to swim?" she sighed.

"I know you have a lot on your plate, but if you can find time to exercise, I predict that your pain will improve. Do you have a friend who can walk with you or join you for a swim class?"

"No, but I used to love to swim. I remember swimming in Sebago Lake as a teenager. We'd jump off the dock and head across the cove." Her eyes brightened. "I could swim forever. Not a care in the world."

"So … it's a good sign that you've been an avid swimmer." This was a positive. Maybe Mrs. Frent can swim her way back to health. I handed her a sheet with the phone numbers of several community pools near her home. She tucked the information into her purse along with a pamphlet on fibromyalgia. I noted that she didn't promise to find time to swim.

"And Lyrica?" she asked. "Could I try a smaller dose than what my doctor prescribed?"

"Yes. Absolutely. Let's limit it to a small nighttime dose. But remember, I almost never see major improvement in fibromyalgia pain with Lyrica unless it's combined with some form of regular exercise as part of the treatment plan."

There was a pause while she retrieved a nearly empty vial of Vicodin from her purse. "And while you're at it, can you refill my Vicodin prescription?"

Thud. Just when I thought the consultation was over, the request for a narcotic took me aback. Despite the fact that no studies have demonstrated their effectiveness in fibromyalgia, narcotics are often prescribed to treat fibromyalgia pain. Faulty reasoning is at the heart of this trend. Fibromyalgia pain is severe. Narcotics are the strongest pain medications we can prescribe. Therefore, narcotics should be effective in fibromyalgia pain. This linkage is untrue; narcotics in fibromyalgia may paradoxically worsen pain by sensitizing the very central nervous system pathways we are trying to block.

To make matters worse, patients like Ms. Frent often experience improvement in pain in the early days and weeks of treatment with narcotics, giving them and their doctor false hope. When the pain worsens, a well-meaning physician may slowly titrate the narcotic dose slowly upward. Over time, though, the pain usually returns full force. The result: some fibromyalgia patients are on high-dose narcotics and still miserable.

I decided to put off her request. "For now, I'd like you to refill your prescription for Vicodin with your primary doctor." We agreed to meet again in a month. Watching her walk down to the checkout counter I was not optimistic.

I was running behind. My next patient was an 80-year-old former Maine fishing guide I followed for osteoporosis. The previous evening, when she attempted to open a stuck window, she felt a sharp *crack* in her back and had spent a restless, painful night in her recliner. When I opened the door to her exam room, the film I ordered on her way in was hanging on the view box. Unfortunately, the fourth vertebrae in the lower spine was clearly fractured. In plain English, she had a broken back.

The woman groaned as she shifted in her chair but was still able to joke, "Can you send me to orthopedics for a new back?"

I silently reviewed her medications and knew that our options were limited. She was already walking daily and on a weekly medication to improve her bone strength. For pain control, she was on high-dose Tylenol and ibuprofen around the clock. Finally, I remembered. "Didn't I prescribe a low dose of Vicodin last year with your first compression fracture?"

"Yes, but I felt woozy and we both worried I might trip, so I stopped it after a few days." She paused. "It *did* help."

Here we were, back-to-back patients with severe pain; one with chronic widespread, *excruciating* soft tissue pain, the other with acute pain from a fracture. In one patient I was certain that prescribing narcotics would be a disservice; in the other, I was bringing up the topic. I pressed firmly at the site of the new compression fracture and asked, "Can you rate how uncomfortable it is where I'm pressing?"

"It's not pleasant. Maybe a 7 on a scale of 1 to 10."

"What do you think about taking half of a Vicodin at night and managing with Tylenol during the day? Oh, and let's see if a twice daily lidocaine patch to your lower back can make you more comfortable while the bone heals." I helped her to her feet and watched as she slowly inched her way to the checkout counter.

On the last day of the month, Mrs. Frent was on the schedule. "I'm still taking the Lyrica at night," she began. "It hasn't helped much with pain but I don't have that fibro fog as much, and I'm sleeping better. I've even had my first visit with a counselor. She's very nice and talks some mumbo jumbo about working on my stressors that are causing problems in my life, and I say, 'Even thinking about stress reduction is stressful.'"

"I'm glad you're seeing the counselor. Stick with it. The swimming? Were you able to sign up for swimming at your local pool?"

"Oh, that's right," she shrugged. "You did mention that. I misplaced the phone number."

"I understand. Here is the number again. Please make time to swim. What else is on your mind?"

"Dr. Wentworth wants to reduce my Vicodin, but it's the only thing that helps my pain. Lately, I've upped it to three times daily and that makes my pain livable, but I'm running out of the pills early. Can you take over the prescription? I don't think Dr. Wentworth understands pain the way you do. He's not a specialist."

Here we go again. I decided to address her request firmly and directly. "No. I won't be picking up the Vicodin prescription. Long-term narcotics do not have a place in the treatment of fibromyalgia. I know it may be difficult for you to accept, but the Vicodin can sensitize the pain pathways in your central nervous system and make your pain worse."

She slumped heavily into her chair. "I knew you wouldn't understand. It's hopeless."

I watched as she trudged out to the checkout counter, and thought this was, most likely, our last office visit. It was not. Over the next two years, Mrs. Frent's pain worsened as her primary care doctor slowly increased the dose of Vicodin. She never did take up my advice to swim or walk regularly. She was up to a half-dozen hydrocodone daily when her doctor called and asked what I thought about switching Mrs. Frent to a longe- acting opioid such as OxyContin. I did not agree with this strategy. By then, we were well into the OxyContin epidemic and not a single study had found that narcotics improved the chronic pain associated with fibromyalgia.

I dreaded our half-hour visits. I simply had nothing new to offer her. At the start of each visit, I would ask Mrs. Frent if her pain was improved, and without exception, she reported that her pain was worse than it was three months before. She experimented with topical and sublingual cannabis preparations and initially reported improved sleep, but eventually drifted away from this as well. Her pain continued to be "excruciating."

Surprisingly, she eventually improved, and it was by accident. She worried about an upcoming move to a rural community an hour from Portland to be closer to her husband's job and family. Even the thought of the move exhausted her. Worse, several weeks before the move, her husband was called away on a long business trip and her son was at camp. There was no one to help. She had no alternative but to ready the house for moving day.

Night after night, after a full day at work, she methodically packed books, lifted chairs, cautiously moved tables, and emptied closets. With the support of her therapist, she stayed in the present, avoiding, as much as possible, the fear of injury. She stretched. She learned to pace her activities. It was hard work. But a curious thing happened. She was so totally exhausted at the end of each day that she collapsed into bed...and slept through the night. Over the next several weeks, her endurance, strength, and pain gradually improved. She was flabbergasted.

At a follow-up visit, I learned that she had signed up for SilverSneakers (a fitness gym for older adults), and took pride in the strength she had gained in her shoulders and low back.

The move to rural Maine was just what she needed. She changed jobs. Her sister-in-law joined her on regular walks. She lost weight. Her son adjusted well to his new school system. Sleep was still an issue, but instead of tossing and turning all night, she awoke most mornings feeling ready to face the day.

Despite the distance, she continued seeing her longtime family doctor, and had decided to work with him on a plan to gradually taper the Vicodin. Over the course of many months, she was able to discontinue it completely. It was hard, sometimes difficult work, but it was worth it.

Chapter 16

"It's far more important to know what person the disease has than what disease the person has." Hippocrates

From the doorway of my office, I watched an elderly man shuffle towards the scale. A blocky rigidity draped over him. His head hung heavily over his chest. Instead of a face, I saw only a mound of shaggy, black unkempt hair. When he stepped cautiously onto the scale, Joanne recorded his weight before the two of them disappeared into an exam room.

I opened Joshua N.'s chart. There was no referral note or X-ray reports. On the front page of the new patient questionnaire he had simply scrawled, *Every morning I wake up my back and knees feel like crap. Ibuprofen is useless. Vicodin helps a little.* The remainder of the questionnaire was blank.

As I closed the chart, I was not under the illusion that I could add much to Joshua N.'s care and hoped that our visit wouldn't focus entirely on narcotics for pain. Hold on. Clear your head, I reprimanded myself. Don't prejudge. There might be quite a lot you can do to improve this poor guy's quality of life. If an X-ray shows that his knees are bone against bone, perhaps I can convince one of the orthopedic surgeons to consider knee replacement.

Physical therapy and soft tissue manipulation might improve his painful back, and there's always the free city pool program. Swimming can build strength and improve balance and reduce pain. Long-term, low-dose opioids? No way. His balance is already impaired, and I'm not going to increase his risk of falling and breaking a hip.

So, I was shocked to enter the exam room and meet Joshua N., *age 22*. The front of his apocalyptic T-shirt pleaded for equality: *Zombies are people too.* "It's okay," he said, noticing the stunned look on my face. "I'm used to the staring. You can call me Josh."

Embarrassed that I had made false assumption after false assumption, I recalibrated and asked Josh when his back problems began.

"First year in high school. I was 14. In the beginning, I thought it was normal." His voice was silky and low, like a jazz radio host. The skin on his cheeks was pockmarked with acne. He shifted slightly and winced, "Do you have a pillow you can put under my butt? Maybe another for my back? Chairs and I don't get along so well."

I reached into a lower cabinet and grabbed two pillows. Josh half-stood and I slid one pillow onto the chair and the other low against the backrest. The faint aroma of onions and garlic and potatoes and gravy permeated the room. He exhaled slowly and continued his story. "So anyway, my mom brought me to our family doctor. The doctor ran a hand up and down my spine and laid me down and cracked my back. Just about killed me. The X-rays showed hardly anything back then—I mean I didn't have this f*ed up, crippled look that I do now. She basically told me to suck it up. I remember her saying, 'Plenty of people have worse problems.' Dirt bag.

"Back then, we lived out a dirt road along the Saco River a couple of miles from Hiram. Midway through eleventh grade I stopped going to school. I didn't lie around; if anything, sitting around makes the pain and stiffness worse. I helped out around the house with my younger brother and sister, learned how to cook, you know, tried to stay busy. Right now, I'm in Portland, working part-time as a short-order cook at the Porthole on the waterfront. I've been living on Motrin. It doesn't help much, but when I run out, especially in the morning, I can barely move."

"Anything else?"

Josh handed me an empty vial of Vicodin. "The medical clinic at Maine Medical Center prescribed these two weeks ago."

"How often are you taking these?" I asked warily.

"A couple at night. I rest better but feel wacky if I take them during the day. Can you refill them? Oh, and I forgot, the clinic took these films and told me to bring them today." From a backpack beneath his seat, Josh pulled out an X-ray folder.

I hung the films on the wall view box. Thick deposits of abnormal bone bridged the space between each vertebra from the base of his skull to his pelvis, forming what radiologists describe as a "bamboo spine." In both hips, only a thin rim of cartilage remained. The diagnosis was unmistakable: ankylosing spondylitis.

At age 22, even if medications could smother the fire of inflammation, there was no resetting the damage. The entire spine was fused in a painful forward flexed position. I placed my stethoscope in my ears to listen to Josh's lungs and heart to settle my mind. It's not often that my emotions disrupt my focus on problem-solving, but even taking away the fact that Josh was 22, his exam and X-rays were the worst I'd ever seen at any age.

"Besides the back," I asked, as if that weren't enough, "are you hurting anywhere else?"

"My knees are killing me. That's been maybe two years. Can you help me roll my pants up? Oh, and my left eye hurts. I went to the emergency room last year and an eye doctor was there treating some kid who got poked in the eye with a pencil. He told me it was iritis--- some weird kind of inflammation— and told me I could go blind if I didn't take care of it. The drops he prescribed really helped, but I've run out and I'm hoping you can refill the prescription."

Now that I noticed, the left eye was slightly puffy and red.

I pulled up Josh's jeans for a better look at his knees. A barbed wire tattoo encircled one calf. Over the mid-shin was a crusty, oozing scab. Both knees were so swollen I was unable to pull the jeans up beyond the mid-calves, so Josh loosened his belt and slipped his jeans down. The sight was gut-wrenching. Each knee held enough fluid to fill a water balloon. I placed one hand on the kneecap and the other on the back of the calf to assess range of motion and Josh reached down and firmly pulled my hand away.

"I'd appreciate it if you just look. Any movement just about sends me through the roof." We sat together for a moment in silence. "Here, let me demonstrate," he said, and flexed the knee ever so slightly. There was an audible clunk. The muscles adjacent to the knee quivered as Josh tried to flex the knee further. The knee joint barely moved.

I was already formulating a plan. Perhaps if we can quiet down the inflammation and have him work intensively with physical therapy his knees and hips can regain normal motion. "Josh, are you okay if I inject the knees with cortisone?"

"I'll try anything once if it can help. Do your worst."

I stuck my head out the door and asked Joanne to set up for an aspiration and injection of each knee. "We'll need multiple 50 cc syringes, two red top and two green top tubes for laboratory testing."

While Joanne set up for the procedures, I returned to my office. Opening a recent journal article on ankylosing spondylitis I was struck once again by the gaps in our understanding of this relatively common disease. For one, why is it that ankylosing spondylitis can be subtle in one patient and cruelly fulminant in another? Why are the sacroiliac joints damaged early in the disease before the inflammation gradually ascends the spine, leading, as in Josh's case, to arthritis of the entire spine. And the disease is not just restricted the spine. Why do many AS patients have eye or bowel inflammation?

Theories on the events leading to ankylosing spondylitis continue to evolve. There is clearly a genetic risk, with roughly 90% of patients positive for the genetic test HLA-B27. On the other hand, the overwhelming majority of people who carry the HLA-B27 gene *never* develop ankylosing spondylitis. What lights the fuse of inflammation in this unfortunate group of patients?

In recent years, researchers have focused on the types of bacteria present in the bowels of patients with ankylosing spondylitis. This emphasis on gut bacteria (the microbiome) and joint inflammation is firmly established in a related disorder called "reactive arthritis" where bacteria such as salmonella or a sexually transmitted infection may trigger joint inflammation several weeks after exposure. Like a hit-and-run accident in which the driver has left the scene, the original infection sometimes can't be identified but has set off chronic inflammation.

But what of ankylosing spondylitis? None of the bacteria implicated in reactive arthritis are chronically present in the bowels of ankylosing spondylitis patients. A host of candidate bacteria have been suggested as triggers but none, as yet, have been conclusively shown to be the cause of the chronic inflammation.

Joanne knocked on the door and told me the injection tray was ready. I reentered Josh's exam room and scrubbed each knee with antiseptic. When I entered the right knee with a 16-gauge needle, there was so much pressure, my syringe filled almost immediately with fluid. Joanne handed me another syringe, then another, and another. Before I was done, I had aspirated four full syringes—200 cc of amber yellow fluid—from each knee. Even after the fluid was aspirated from the knees and I injected them with steroids, Josh could barely flex and extend the knees. For the first time in my practice career, I decided to admit a 22-year-old patient for inflammatory arthritis.

After office hours, on my drive to the hospital, I recalled a rheumatology colleague of mine, Muhammad Asim Khan, MD, who first developed symptoms of ankylosing spondylitis at the age of twelve. Despite the limitations and rapid progression of his disease, he graduated from medical school and became a rheumatologist. Over the years I would often see Dr. Khan at national rheumatology meetings. When a fellow rheumatologist called out his name, he smiled and turned, his feet shuffling towards the greeting as the lower spine and neck and head moved en bloc. In a spine transformed by inflammation and damage, his smile was radiant, his spirit somehow unbowed.

I stopped by the hospital after hours and Josh was asleep in bed, curled up on his side, his hair neatly combed, the *Zombies are people too!* T-shirt replaced by a hospital gown. I reviewed the physical and occupational therapy initial progress notes and wrote a series of orders to follow through on several of their recommendations. Despite some misgivings, I continued his nighttime dose of hydrocodone.

I considered my next step, an infusion of Remicade, the new medication Ben Shipman, my RA patient from Chebeague Island, had recently responded to in our office research study. Now that it was approved by the FDA for both rheumatoid arthritis and ankylosing spondylitis, recent studies suggested that in some patients, regular infusions of TNF blockers could slow down or prevent progression of ankylosing spondylitis.

But as a potent immune suppressant, the drug was not for everyone. Patients can develop serious, sometimes life-threatening infections during treatment. Observing Josh while he slept, I noted that there were no needle marks on his hands or forearms. That's all we need, I thought. If he's an IV drug user, aggressively treating him with Remicade will be a disaster. Josh stirred and I sat down at the bedside to explain ankylosing spondylitis in terms that he could make sense of. Despite dropping out of school, he had a good grasp of the basics and was open to "anything that can help."

Later that night, motoring across to Peaks Island on a cool, windless summer night, a quote from Thomas Wolfe came to mind: "Man is born to live, to suffer, and to die, and what befalls him is a tragic lot. There is no denying this in the final end. But we must deny it all along the way." But what if the suffering is unremitting day and night, month after month, year after year? How can one make peace with this level of suffering? Or more specifically, how had rheumatologist Muhammad Khan, MD somehow adapted to his chronic pain and limitations?

Abraham Verghese, MD, a Professor of Medicine at Stanford University, has said that in his former practice in rural Tennessee working with HIV patients (at a time when there was no effective treatment for HIV) he learned the critical difference between healing and curing. "One can be healed only when there is no cure, by which I mean a coming to terms with the illness, finding some level of peace and acceptance in such a terrible setting."

Andrew Still, DO, the founder of osteopathic medicine, recognized that the vital forces of the body are its greatest healers. The physician's role in chronic illness is to gently turn our patients away from self-pity, anger, and destructive behaviors. Physicians, even when they cannot cure, can make the journey a little easier. After tying off SAKAMO at my float shortly before midnight, I walked slowly home. Off to the east a shimmering curtain of lights played on the horizon. Bands of pink and blue radiated towards the Orion constellation in the moonless sky. Arriving home, I awakened Sandi and we stood quietly outside as the Northern Lights spread along the horizon. And then, as mysteriously as the lights appeared, they faded away. Back inside, we peeked into Kate and Molly's bedrooms as they slumbered. What emotional and physical traumas will they face? Can a parent teach resiliency?

Nursing called at 2 a.m. "Your patient is rating his pain as an 8 on a scale of 1 to 10. You don't have any orders for additional hydrocodone," the nurse said brusquely. "Do you want to change that to an every-four-hour order?"

"I won't be ordering additional narcotics for breakthrough pain." I had an uneasy feeling about Josh. I knew so little about him.

"Fine." There was an awkward silence, then she added, "He's here, in part, for better control of his pain, isn't he?"

"Yes, but this isn't like postsurgical pain. I'm not going to liberalize Josh's narcotics based on the number 8. We're going to manage his pain with anti-inflammatories, Remicade, intravenous steroids, and physical therapy. Let's see how he's doing tomorrow."

There was a heavy silence on the other end. I had the feeling that the nurse was writing down some type of incident report or complaint against me. I wasn't in the mood to discuss my approach to Josh's chronic pain and ended the conversation with, "...and please don't call the on-call medicine resident tonight for additional pain meds."

The hospitalization was of some benefit. On the plus side, Josh's knees were significantly better after the cortisone injections and physical therapy, and his back pain was reduced by perhaps fifty percent. His eye inflammation resolved and his vision returned to normal. He no longer required a cane.

But there were plenty of negatives. Because the bones in Josh's neck and back were fused, he remained stooped and lacked, what rheumatologists call horizon vision. His eyes focused on his feet. I asked an orthopedic colleague for a consult on Josh's damaged hips and knees. He agreed that joint replacement could be considered, but we should delay this as long as possible. If at age 22 Josh underwent joint replacements, he would undoubtedly require additional surgery before age 40, and revisions of joint replacements are notoriously complex and difficult.

I knew that we were dealing with a particularly aggressive form of ankylosing spondylitis when I saw Josh in the office only two weeks after his discharge and the fluid in his knees had reaccumulated, and the markers of inflammation—ESR and CRP—were nearly back to their pre-hospitalization levels. I increased the dose of Remicade for the next infusion and once again injected the knees.

In the ensuing weeks and months, Josh's disease slowly came under some semblance of control. He continued his part-time job as a short-order cook but pain management became more and more problematic. From time to time, he called for early refills on his hydrocodone and on one occasion, claimed that his pills were ruined when the top of his prescription vial came off and the pills were soaked in the rain. I stood firm; refilling his prescription early was out of the question, and I began to worry, was he diverting the narcotics for cash and supplementing his income? He missed one office appointment, and then another.

But Josh always showed for his monthly infusion of Remicade. Relaxing in a recliner upstairs at our infusion center and chatting away with his new friend, lobsterman Ben Shipman, he seemed to accept membership in a club no one wants to join, the doing better, but still nearly disabled club.

Josh continued to smoke, a clear risk factor for infection on immune suppressants. A year after our first visit I admitted Josh with fulminant pneumonia, his oxygen levels so low, he was nearly placed on a ventilator. By day four, however, he was on the mend and out of the intensive care unit. On my way into the hospital several days after he was transferred to the general floor and off oxygen, I watched Josh wheel an IV pole outside to the designated smoking area and light up. Like an angry parent, I crossed the street and chewed him out. Josh admitted that smoking was probably not the best way to celebrate his first day off oxygen, but it helped him relax. He was *thinking* about quitting.

Phraseology matters: *Thinking about quitting* is a world away from *I've set a date, I am quitting.* His addiction to smoking while struggling to breathe did not bode well for remaining on the Remicade. Out of safety concerns, I held his Remicade for a month, and the ankylosing spondylitis promptly flared. More injections in the knees followed. Back on track with an infusion of Remicade, his disease improved once more.

At some point, Josh stopped coming to the office and was a no-show for several Remicade infusions. I suspected that he had transitioned into an addict. We never had been able to eliminate the nighttime hydrocodone. I checked the obituaries in the paper. Joanne finally tracked down a number for Josh's mother, who was living with a sister outside of Portland. I called her after hours.

"Josh is in jail," she said. "Dealing drugs. They got him and now he's in the Thomaston Prison." There was a long pause. "I only hope they give him a break. That boy has suffered enough."

As the years went by, I often thought of Josh. Had he been released from prison? For that matter, was he still alive? If alive, had he undergone hip or knee replacement? At our weekly rheumatology conference, Josh's name would come up, as in, this patient has very active, progressive disease, but not as severe as Josh N"s ankylosing spondylitis. The other rheumatologists would nod their heads in agreement. His was the worst case of inflammatory arthritis anyone in our office had ever treated. The absolute worst.

One late-summer morning, I watched from my office doorway as Joanne guided Josh down the hallway to the scale, his gait smoother than I'd remembered. She brought him into an exam room, and as I walked by the half-open door, he was settled in a cushioned chair, one pillow accommodating his back, the other beneath his butt. A floral bowling shirt hung loosely over jeans.

Settling into an adjacent chair, I scanned his front pocket: no cigarettes. Good. On his feet he wore bowling shoes with a Velcro strap closure. Very classy.

"It's great to see you Josh," I began. I ran a finger down his list of medications. "I see that the prison doctor switched you from the IV infusions of Remicade to a weekly shot of Enbrel. Is that working for you?"

"Well enough." He shifted in his chair so that he could see my face and pointed to my hearing aids and glasses. "Hey, you're getting old." Then Josh dropped his trousers so that I could examine his matching knee and hip replacements.

The prison doctor had taken good care of him. When Josh reached a point where he could no longer walk on his damaged hips and knees, he referred him to an orthopedic surgeon in nearby Camden, who replaced his hips. A year later, he tackled the knees. The joint replacements functioned well.

During his years of incarceration, Josh had earned his GED, and now worked at a local vegetarian restaurant. His old girlfriend (they'd gotten together again after he was released from prison) was sharing an apartment with him. "Next week, I'm getting a raise. I'll be responsible for scheduling the line cooks and dishwashers in the kitchen. I'm no longer a line cook." He raised an amused eyebrow. "Call me Mr. Chef."

I scratched my cheek, waiting. I was wary. If Josh was after narcotics, I was prepared to say no. I had been burned so many times. But Josh had other ideas. He handed me a copy of a medical journal article on spinal surgery in ankylosing spondylitis patients. "You probably know about this, but they break your back in multiple places and take a wedge out of each vertebra. Then they put in some rods and screws, well, maybe more than a few rods and screws, and straighten the back. After the surgery, I'll look more like a normal person instead of a bum staring at his shoes. What do you think?"

I knew what Josh was referring to. It was a massive, complex surgery. Only specialized centers with highly experienced spine surgeons were willing to take apart a fused bamboo spine and put it back together. The risk of infection, bleeding, hardware loosening, or even paralysis was high. Following the surgery, Josh would go through months of painful rehab. There was a risk that he could be worse off than he was now, even die from complications of surgery. And there was another obstacle; there was no guarantee that a surgeon would take him on.

“You sure you want to start down this road?” I asked.

“Positive.” Josh stood; his eyes locked onto his shoes. “I know where I’ve been. I just want to see where I’m going. That’s not too much to ask, is it?”

I began the paperwork.

Chapter 17

"Not every doctor works for every patient."
Ron Anderson, MD

Outside the exam room, I leaned against the wall and shut my eyes. There was no way forward. At its core, Mr. Jewell has a belief system that is contradictory to mine. We belong to different religions, each hoping to convince the other to convert. I am the establishment, unwilling to adopt the long-term antibiotic approach for Lyme disease he has embraced as an article of faith.

An hour earlier, I had asked Joanne, "Any referral notes or laboratory studies for me to review ahead of time on my new patient?"

"No, he'd prefer to tell you the story from the beginning. Fresh."

"Okay," I said, the inflection in my voice indicating otherwise. "Did he fill out the new patient questionnaire?"

"No," Joanne raised an eyebrow. "He has his records organized in a 3-ring binder. Good luck."

"Thanks." I lingered outside the exam room. When a patient brings their own records, it usually means that multiple consultants have seen the patient. Having it fed to me selectively, page by page, makes it clear that the patient disagrees with some or all of the previous opinions. Lab or radiographic studies may be conflicting. Medications have been either ineffective or poorly tolerated. I am about to hear a medical journey from a particular viewpoint. "Did you notice anything when you roomed him?"

"He was limping," Joanne answered. "Maybe a bad knee?"

"Okay, that's a start." I felt at a distinct disadvantage not knowing anything about my next consult, even mildly irritated. Based on my previous experiences, this next hour may not go well for either of us. Careful, I reminded myself. He's a patient who needs help. Don't prejudge. Clear your mind; the man is limping.

I extended my hand as I entered the room. "Good morning Mr. Jewell."

"Good morning. Thank you for seeing me. Let me start at the beginning, two years ago when I first developed Lyme disease." Mr. Jewell cracked open the notebook as if he were reading a bedtime story. "My property is infested with ticks; it's overrun with ticks. I'm constantly pulling them off the dogs, but one evening, I found an embedded tick on my lower leg and it was quite a process to remove it. Well, I went to the doctor and showed her the remains."

With this, Mr. Jewell handed me a test tube as he repositioned his black-framed glasses on the bridge of his nose. "As you can see, it was a deer tick, not the larger, innocuous dog tick." I held the tube up to the light and identified a mummified dark spot the size of a grain of rice nestled on a wad of cotton. Mr. Jewell turned to the next page labeled: TREATMENT. "The doctor prescribed doxycycline. That would be August 24th. Two hundred mg of doxycycline."

"And did that help?" I asked, before noticing a line of oily grime around the cuff of my trouser leg. That would be from when I stepped into my boat an hour ago and water from a recent thunderstorm flooded over my shoe. My left foot still felt uncomfortably cold. On my tie was a gray smudge—probably from when I leaned down to inspect the bilge pump. I tucked the tie into my shirt.

"Evidently not." Mr. Jewell hiked up his slacks for me to view his swollen knee. "Can you imagine, two pills of 100 mg doxycycline? What was the doctor thinking?"

I recalled that the Center for Disease Control recommendation for prevention of Lyme disease after pulling off an embedded tick was indeed 200 mg of doxycycline. At a glance, I estimated that Mr. Jewell's knee held half a cup of fluid. No wonder he was limping, an effusion that large must be painful. Above the knee I glimpsed a silvery, quarter-sized rash on the inner thigh, but as I leaned forward to get a better look, Mr. Jewell tugged his pants cuff down several inches.

"There's a large amount of fluid in this knee," I said. "Has it ever been tapped?"

"Once. But we're getting ahead of ourselves." Mr. Jewell grimaced as he shifted the knee and turned the page. "After the tick bite I didn't notice much. I'd heard about Lyme disease, everyone's heard about Lyme disease, but it wasn't until the following spring when the Lyme symptoms began. At first, I thought it was the divorce. I wasn't sleeping well and I've always been prone to headaches, but every day, my head throbbed. I gained weight." He patted his abdomen as if to emphasize the obvious. “At work, I was so exhausted I could hardly drag myself back to the office after lunch.”

“And when did the knee swelling occur?” I asked.

“Out of nowhere the knee swelled up one month later.”

“And did someone see you for that?”

“An orthopedic surgeon.” Mr. Jewell removed several pages from his records and handed them to me. I scanned through the results: normal X-ray, negative Lyme testing, and handed them back. “At the end of the visit, he injected the knee with cortisone.”

“And did that help?” I asked.

“It was amazing. Complete relief. But in retrospect, that was probably the worst thing he could have done. I’m sure you’re aware that injecting a Lyme-infected knee with cortisone allows the infection free reign. When the swelling relapsed several months later, I felt like someone had exploded a bomb inside it. That’s when I heard about Dr. Finegold, a Lyme-savvy doctor in Massachusetts. He was a godsend.”

“That would be, what, a year ago?” I asked.

“Yes.” Mr. Jewell handed me another two pages. “Here’s his consult. I was a train wreck by then. Although a second Lyme test was negative, Dr. Finegold assured me that the negative Lyme testing represented a false negative, probably related to the inadequate initial treatment of the imbedded tick the previous year. He emphasized that Lyme is a clinical diagnosis. Testing is notoriously iffy. No, I don’t think he used the word iffy, but you know what I mean, the symptoms, the big picture, that’s what he was looking at to make the diagnosis of chronic Lyme disease. Dr. Finegold had me fill out a Lyme disease questionnaire. You’ll notice that I checked off 32 out of 42 symptoms commonly associated with Lyme disease.”

Indeed. Included in the checklist suggesting Lyme disease was *#28: Disturbed sleep: too much, too little,* and *#40: Exaggerated symptoms or worse hangover from alcohol.*

"Dr. Finegold cautioned me that I was one of the worst cases he'd ever seen and that treatment would require a multifaceted approach. Even so, he was optimistic that a full recovery was possible, even expected. So, for three months I took doxycycline. After that, well, we tried different combinations of oral antibiotics and supplements. The swelling in the knee didn't budge. The theory, well, I'm sure you already know this, but the Lyme spirochete is capable of evading the immune system. That's when he arranged for a month of the intravenous antibiotic, let me make sure I say this right, Ceftriaxone."

My head was spinning. An embedded tick promptly treated with the appropriate dose of doxycycline, two negative Lyme tests, months of oral antibiotics and now a course of intravenous antibiotics. Lyme arthritis? I don't think so. Something else must be driving the knee inflammation.

"There were times during the first four months of antibiotic treatment that I believed I was turning the corner, but then almost overnight, the pain and swelling in my knee doubled. The tick was fighting back. My short-term memory was shot; my mood swings horrific. And the fatigue…I could barely will myself out of bed each morning. I was losing the battle. When my arm veins could no longer be used, Dr. Finegold recommended that I have a port placed."

Mr. Jewell reached up to his upper left chest where the port was palpable beneath the skin (through the port, medications can be delivered directly into a large vein). "Once the port was in, Dr. Finegold doubled the dose of the IV antibiotics. It was a last-ditch effort, but it wasn't enough. I lost my job and applied for disability —that would be four months ago."

"I'm sorry it came to that." I forced a tight-lipped half smile, stood and unfolded a cloth gown from the shelf above the sink. "Let me step out for a minute while you change into a gown. I want to do a complete examination. I'll be back in a few minutes."

Back in my office I slumped into my swivel chair and pulled a review article on Lyme disease from my files. In the mid-1970s, two young mothers from Lyme, Connecticut, Polly Murray and Judith Mensch, contacted their State Health Department. Both had children that had been diagnosed with JIA (juvenile idiopathic arthritis), and they knew of other children and adults with similar symptoms. Since JIA is an uncommon immune system disease affecting about 1 in 1000 children, and the mothers' story suggested far higher numbers, Dr. Allen Steere, a first-year fellow in rheumatology, and Dr. Stephen Malawista, the head of the rheumatology department at Yale New Haven Hospital, decided to investigate the unusual cluster.

With the mothers' assistance, the two physicians eventually identified 39 children with the disorder in the surrounding community. Many of the families recalled that their child developed a flu-like illness and an unusual rash before experiencing joint swelling. Steere and Malawista reported their findings in the Journal of Arthritis and Rheumatism: *Lyme Arthritis: An Epidemic of Oligoarticular Arthritis in Children and Adults in Three Connecticut Communities.*

By the time I arrived at Yale New Haven Hospital as a visiting internal medicine resident for a six-month elective in 1984, many of the details of Lyme disease had been clarified. A bacterium, *Borrelia burgdorferi,* transmitted by the bite of the deer tick, was determined to be the cause of Lyme disease. An expanding rash (erythema migrans) occurred in many, but not all patients after the initial tick bite, and represented the leading edge of the infection.

In untreated patients, a flu-like illness with fevers, muscle and joint aching, and fatigue developed. In patients promptly treated with antibiotics, the infection usually resolved. And there were other, more serious complications. Unrecognized Lyme infection could lead to heart rhythm disturbances or inflammation within the central nervous system (meningitis) as well as peripheral nerve damage. Some patients eventually developed inflammatory arthritis, usually in a solitary joint such as the knee, but occasionally in smaller joints.

Even though Yale was a hotbed of Lyme research, in our rheumatology clinics, we didn't automatically assume that all of our patients with swollen joints or unexplained symptoms had Lyme arthritis. After all, there are nearly 100 conditions rheumatologists treat, and Lyme disease was only one of many possibilities. Even in challenging cases, however, clues in the history or physical exam and laboratory studies usually led to a specific diagnosis. Sometimes, it was Lyme disease.

Now, decades later, I'm relieved when Lyme testing is positive in my inflammatory arthritis patients. Instead of having a chronic, lifelong disease, they have an infection that is usually cured by a month of the oral antibiotic doxycycline, or, in some resistant cases, a month of intravenous Ceftriaxone.

Of course, nothing in medicine is simple; there *are* exceptions.

As our understanding of Lyme arthritis has expanded, a number of studies (including papers written by Dr. Steere), have suggested that rarely, the Lyme spirochete may trigger persistent joint inflammation despite appropriate antibiotics, a process called "reactive arthritis." That is, the original infection has resolved, but swelling and inflammation persists due to activation of the immune system. These patients respond well to medications which reduce inflammation.

Returning to Mr. Jewell's room, I noticed that three fingernails had distinctive tiny pits and asked, "Have you noticed the changes in your nails?"

"I have," he replied. "I keep discovering that the Lyme is hanging on in places I wouldn't dream of. It's not just the fluid in the knee. Dr. Finegold said that I'd know when the Lyme infection was on the run when the nails began to heal."

I continued my exam. A silvery patch of skin over the back of the right elbow caught my attention. Psoriasis. Above the knee, the silvery patch of skin in the mid-thigh I'd glimpsed earlier was also definitely psoriasis. On a hunch, I asked him to slip off his shoes and socks, and here was another clue. The third toe on the right foot was reddened and swollen like a sausage.

An alternative explanation for his joint symptoms was clearly present. The skin psoriasis and pitted nails, the swollen knee and inflamed toe represented psoriatic arthritis, not Lyme arthritis. Nothing else fit. For more than a year, Mr. Jewell had suffered unnecessarily and was now applying for disability with both the wrong diagnosis and on the wrong treatment.

"I've been off the infusions for several months," Mr. Jewell interrupted my thoughts, "ever since my insurance company refused to cover them."

Now I understood why Mr. Jewell was in my office selectively feeding me his medical records. In essence, his health insurance company was asking: *Do you agree with Mr. Jewell's treatment with long-term IV antibiotics for Lyme arthritis?*

Intravenous infusions are not only expensive, running into thousands of dollars per month, but are associated with significant risks, including allergic reactions, systemic infections, and in rare cases, death.

After completing my exam, I asked Mr. Jewell to change and slowly walked back to my office. There, I cracked open a pistachio nut and considered my strategy. How do I convince Mr. Jewell that he has psoriatic arthritis, not Lyme arthritis? Then I sat quietly for a moment, recalling the fractious history of Lyme disease.

Following the development of antibiotic treatment regimens for Lyme disease in the 1980s, it became clear that while most patients with Lyme disease promptly recovered, approximately one in ten experienced persistent and at times life-altering fatigue, headaches, and migratory muscle and joint pain. The term, *post-Lyme disease syndrome*, was coined to describe this patient subgroup. Because academic researchers could not identify persistent infection, antibiotics were not recommended for this group of patients. Although most of these patients eventually recovered, a significant number remained unwell.

Advocacy and support groups were formed to promote an alternative view: Patient's symptoms continued because the original infection was present within cells and difficult, if not impossible, to detect. The diagnosis of *Chronic Lyme disease* came into the popular lexicon.

The two sides disagreed on nearly every aspect of Lyme disease, including how often Lyme testing was negative in Lyme disease, antibiotic dosing for prevention of Lyme disease after an embedded tick, and duration of antibiotic treatment for chronic Lyme disease. Eventually, because they remained unwell, patients like Mr. Jewell not uncommonly received long-term IV antibiotics through a port.

But does this approach work?

To answer this question, researchers designed a study to compare placebo infusions with IV antibiotics in patients with persistent symptoms after a diagnosis of Lyme disease. Four separate studies failed to show that IV antibiotics were more effective than a placebo infusion. This did not end the controversy. As described in David Grann's 2001 article in The New York Times Magazine, *Stalking Dr. Steere*, "The Lyme movement considered itself a victim of...(the) scientific establishment...It formed its own powerful organizations, such as the Lyme Disease Foundation, created its own scientific publication, the *Journal of Spirochetal and Tick-Borne Diseases,* organized its own scientific conferences, and trumpeted its own medical experts with their own treatments."

What's more, the dispute became intensely personal. Dr. Steere, who had originally described the tick-born infection and did not recommend long-term antibiotics, at one point required security guards at his scientific lectures. Official complaints were lodged against him at the state medical licensing board. These were found to be without merit.

Mr. Jewell's case was even more mind-boggling.

There was no question in my mind that his knee inflammation and rash represented psoriatic arthritis. His Lyme testing had never been positive and the myriad symptoms he had checked off on his Lyme disease questionnaire overlapped with symptoms in patients with a host of other painful medical conditions, including untreated psoriatic arthritis.

Joanne knocked on my office door and whispered, "You're running behind. Lynn P. is in room #3. Can you see her before you finish up your consult with Mr. Jewell? She's three months pregnant and needs to pick up her son from first grade."

"Pregnant?" The welcome news turned my morning around. "How is she?"

"She's doing just fine," Joanne answered. "Her RA flared when you stopped her methotrexate a few months before she became pregnant [methotrexate increases the risk of birth defects]. The low-dose prednisone you began over the phone controlled her joint inflammation. Last week was her first visit with her obstetrician, Dr. Rolandelli, and the three-month ultrasound of the baby was normal."

Inside the exam room, Lynn was absolutely beaming. Although her wrists were slightly tender, her grip was excellent and there was no evidence for inflammation elsewhere. Even more amazing, in recent weeks, she had recently been able to discontinue prednisone and her joints remained comfortable. This common but poorly understood phenomenon, rheumatoid arthritis remission during pregnancy, does not occur in all patients but when it does, patients (and their doctors) are overjoyed. Unfortunately, as mysteriously as RA improves during pregnancy, it invariably relapses in the weeks and months after delivery.

Then I recalled that Dr. Rolandelli was not only a skilled obstetrician, but to pass the time during labor and delivery, he knitted caps for his newborn babies. His office bulletin board was awash with photos of babies wearing their first Maine wool caps. "Do you know what color cap Dr. Rolandelli is planning to knit?" I asked.

"We can't be sure yet if it's a girl or a boy. I have another ultrasound in two months. Sometimes boys hide," Lynn teased me.

The visit reset my day. After all Lynn P. had gone through, she was experiencing an uneventful pregnancy off of all medications. I recalled Professor Andy Balber's introductory immunology class at Bates College. If he were teaching the class today, almost certainly the puzzle of why RA often goes into remission during pregnancy would have been one of his memorable blank slides.

Returning to Mr. Jewell's room, and aware that I was hopelessly behind schedule, I saw no reason to delay or hedge on my opinion. From past experience, I suspected this was not going to go well. "I have some good news for you, Mr. Jewell. It may take a few months, but with some medication adjustments, I believe that the pain and swelling in your knee can be dramatically improved. Instead of Lyme arthritis, you have psoriatic arthritis, a very treatable condition."

For a moment, there was stunned silence. Then Mr. Jewell's face collapsed and he looked like he was on the verge of tears. One would have thought that I had diagnosed him with an incurable malignancy. "I knew it," he hung his head. "My sister said I should come see you, but this is exactly what I expected." He gathered his notebook and jacket and stood to leave. I cracked my neck to the right and surreptitiously palpated my pulse. That's strange. I'm sweating like crazy and about to ignite from stress and my pulse is a rock-steady 60 per minute. Go figure. The human body is a strange mixture of mind-body interactions. Some make sense, some do not.

"Here, let me explain." I pulled a dermatology textbook from the shelf and opened it to photos of skin psoriasis. Mr. Jewell reluctantly sat down for a better look. "I think you can agree that your skin rashes represent psoriasis. Roughly 20% of patients with skin psoriasis also have inflamed joints, what we call psoriatic arthritis. Since there is no specific blood test to confirm a diagnosis of psoriatic arthritis, my job is to weigh the evidence between a diagnosis of psoriatic arthritis and other forms of inflammatory arthritis and recommend a course of treatment."

Mr. Jewell considered this. "So, you agree with Dr. Finegold?"

"No. My opinion is that you have psoriatic arthritis and don't need further antibiotics." I wasn't going to leave any wiggle room in our discussion.

"What about the Lyme diagnostic questionnaire?"

"The questionnaire? It's not specific for Lyme disease. If any of my patients with active psoriatic or rheumatoid arthritis filled out the questionnaire, it's likely their answers would be similar to yours." I paused. Mr. Jewell seemed to be mulling over my logic.

"Then why do I feel better when I'm on IV antibiotics?" he asked finally.

"There are many reasons why symptoms of fatigue or concentration or pain may feel better with a treatment you and your doctor believe in. But remember, I'm saying *symptoms*. Your knee swelling is a sign, a measurable objective finding. I don't see where that has improved with intravenous antibiotics. Has it?"

He glumly looked at his knee. "I'm not sure. Sometimes I think it's getting better. Dr. Finegold has repeatedly told me that treatment of my arthritis is going to take time. If only the diagnosis of Lyme disease hadn't been delayed so long, I'd probably be back to normal."

I was anything if not persistent. "Look at how much you've declined during the past year despite antibiotics," I countered. "A year ago, you didn't need a cane to walk. Six months ago, you were working. Going forward, if you allow me to treat you for psoriatic arthritis, I'm confident that we can control the inflammation and prevent future damage."

Mr. Jewell rubbed his knee and flexed it slowly back and forth. "What type of medication are you suggesting?"

“Okay. In order to achieve our goal of putting your psoriatic arthritis in remission, I want to begin a weekly medication called methotrexate. It’s an older but very effective drug, so we know a lot about how it works, the risks, and the proven benefits.” As I talked, I noticed Mr. Jewell typing on his iPhone. “And although we need to monitor it for side effects with blood counts and liver testing, the knee swelling should respond…”

“It says here…” Mr. Jewell interrupted me. “It says here, that methotrexate is a drug that is used in chemotherapy. It’s an immunosuppressant, a cancer drug.”

“That’s true.” I swallowed and fought back the urge to escalate the conversation. “Yes, its original use was in cancer medicine, but the dose of methotrexate we use in psoriatic arthritis is a fraction of the dose used in chemotherapy. In the proper dose, it’s well tolerated and helps reset an overactive and misdirected immune system without suppressing it. Some of my patients have safely taken methotrexate for decades. If the methotrexate doesn’t fully control the inflammation, a new class of medications, biologic response modifiers such as Enbrel or Remicade—and there are others—are often remarkably effective in the management of psoriatic arthritis.”

Mr. Jewell crossed his arms and looked beyond me at the clock. Both of us needed a time-out. “Hold tight,” I said’ “I’ll be back in a moment.” I walked slowly down the hallway to the bathroom, poured myself a cup of coffee in the break room, drank half of it, and poured the rest in the sink. Then I returned to Mr. Jewell’s exam room. “Okay, now where were we?”

“We were talking about medications,” Mr. Jewell replied.

“Right. And I assume you’ve had a chance to read more about methotrexate?”

"I have. And I would never take a drug like methotrexate or any of the other medications you've suggested. Dr. Finegold has a plan. He's explained to me that the Lyme infection hides out inside our cells. It's constantly changing and evolving. That's why I need to bathe my system with combinations of antibiotics, to catch it when it emerges. My immune system needs help. We need to build it up with supplements and changes in diet and you're asking me to ingest a drug that will tear down my immune system and poison my liver."

Checkmate. There was no room for compromise.

"Then I guess we'll need to agree to disagree. I'm sorry that so far, your inflammatory arthritis, what I'm calling psoriatic arthritis, hasn't responded to what Dr. Finegold has prescribed for Lyme disease. I'll summarize my thoughts to your primary care doctor and leave the door open to see you in the future. If you change your mind, I can…"

"That's fine, except for one thing," Mr. Jewell leaned forward on his seat. "I need a letter so that I can restart the IV antibiotics through my port. My insurance company is pressuring me to stop the antibiotics, and I need the form filled out and signed by a rheumatologist."

Stone-faced, I chewed on my inner lip. "No," I said finally. "I'm not willing to do that. I don't agree with your treatment plan." The visit was over. I don't recall what Mr. Jewell said as he gathered his belongings and stormed out. The limp was real. His disease was real, only it was the wrong disease. Sometimes in life, we pick the wrong door.

Chapter 18

Six weeks with a fever is an eternity.
— Honoré de Balzac
Attributed as a conversation on his death bed with his doctor.

I have no idea what's wrong with Mrs. Nash.

She is an FUO, medical parlance for a "fever of unknown origin" patient, and the trigger for her mysterious illness has remained elusive despite four months of extensive testing. One morning she might be pain free, and the next, her knuckles would swell to the point she couldn't make a fist. Increasingly, she needed her husband's help with simple tasks: buttoning her clothes, pulling up a zipper, using a knife to cut her food.

I am in good company. Rheumatologist Ron Anderson at Brigham and Women's Hospital in Boston once confided to a surprised group of medical students on medical rounds, "That disease saw me a long time before I saw it," meaning, even experienced clinicians at world-class institutions are sometimes stumped.

The previous spring, when I met Mrs. Nash for the first time, there was no indication that she was in the early stages of a mysterious illness. Through the partially open door of my office, I watched Joanne lead her into an exam room, her silver white hair offset by a gray cashmere sweater and ankle length skirt. She was stocky but not obese. A rubbery squeak on the linoleum floor punctuated each step from her L.L. Bean boots.

As I reviewed her family doctor's referral notes, her case initially appeared to be straightforward. Mrs. Nash was 68 years old, married, with four adult children and eleven grandchildren. She was, remarkably, on no prescription medications. A single line summarized her past medical history: diet-controlled diabetes. The second page provided me with details of her recent illness. Following a sore throat and cough, she had developed generalized muscle aching and stiffness in the wrists and fingers. Her doctor had handwritten in the margin: *Patient miserable. Cough resolved but joint and muscle pain keeping her awake at night. Low-grade fevers persist. Post-viral syndrome?* And I thought to myself, *that sounds entirely reasonable.* This should not take long; residual fatigue and muscle and joint pain is not unusual after a viral illness. It should burn out.

Then I opened the door and Mrs. Nash reached into her purse and pulled out a notebook of hand-written notes. "Thank you for seeing me. I'm a mess and don't know where to start."

"Well, let's begin with the last time you were well." I exhaled slowly, resetting my expectations. This will take some time.

She ran a finger down the left side of the first page. "March 14th. Larry, my husband, kept me up all night with a nasty cough. Later that same week, I was coughing too."

I glanced down at the last name on her chart. Of course, now I remembered; Larry Nash DO, a retired general surgeon, was her husband. Her family doctor, Dr. Hanson, had called me earlier in the week hoping I could fit her in. Hmm, that rules out lunch. Emergent spousal consults generally fall into two distinct categories; both take a long time. Either there is hypervigilance regarding persistent but innocent symptoms, or the patient has a rare, life-threatening disorder. In rheumatology, there seems to be no middle ground. Mrs. Nash, based on her healthy appearance and attention to detail, had a heavy dose of the former.

"By March 24th, Larry was fine, he bounced back, but I took a turn for the worse. Stiff? I was so stiff I could hardly move. That's when we decided I should see Dr. Hanson."

"And I have his notes here." Filling in the blanks, I've learned, helps consolidate the story and also lets the patient know that I've reviewed their chart. "Your chest X-ray was normal, and the basic lab was normal as well."

"Well, not really." She pointed to one of the laboratory studies in her referral letter where the BUN (blood urea nitrogen) was one point above the normal range.

I blinked before answering. "The BUN, yes the BUN is borderline, but with the other kidney test very much in the normal range, the BUN doesn't have any significance."

"That's what my husband, Larry, thought," she replied. "But it's not normal." I am thinking: *precise, literal, use language carefully.* She turned to the next page. "So anyway, Dr. Hanson thought it was probably a virus but since my cough was hanging on and he couldn't rule out a bacterial infection, he prescribed an antibiotic, azithromycin."

"And?" I asked.

"It didn't work. I'm worse. Much worse."

As we talked, I methodically examined Mrs. Nash's joints, lungs, heart, skin, neck, and abdomen. Normal. Normal. Normal. My thought process shifted to *how can I reassure Mrs. Nash that she's going to be just fine...*

"Lately, I'm sweating at night. Not every night. After midnight, on April 12th, 18th, and the 21st, I soaked the bed and had to change my nightclothes. And fevers? I've kept a graph." She handed me a meticulously diagrammed chart where her temperature was recorded. During the day, the temperatures were in the normal range, but each evening Mrs. Nash spiked a fever of 103, sometimes 104 degrees.

Abruptly, the dynamics of the visit had changed; night sweats and fevers five weeks into an apparent viral infection suggest a serious illness. I stuck my head out the exam door and asked Joanne to inform my next patient that I was running late. I wondered if I still had some salted cashews or a bag of Doritos in my office.

After finishing my exam, I told Mrs. Nash that while her symptoms might represent a persistent viral infection, we needed to run further studies. "I know your chest X-ray was normal, but with the night sweats…"

"Larry thought you might want to get a CT scan of the chest and abdomen."

"Right. So, let's get you scheduled for that," I said without skipping a beat. Though Dr. Nash was not in the room, he seemed to be very much present in our deliberations. "I'm also adding some immunologic laboratory tests and a set of blood cultures. We'll need a urine sample. I'd like you to take a prescription for daily meloxicam, a relative of ibuprofen. It may help quiet down your muscle aching and joint pain."

"Anything except prednisone," her voice sharpened. "I once had an asthma attack and the emergency room doctor gave me a prescription for prednisone. I couldn't sleep for a week and my blood sugars went through the roof. And in case it's not listed in my medical records, I have osteopenia. My bones are brittle enough without adding prednisone, thank you." With that, she glanced at her watch, closed the notebook and gathered her purse. In another moment, she was gone.

Later that day, I reviewed Mrs. Nash's preliminary results. Circled in red, her elevated inflammatory markers laid to rest any notion that she was on the tail end of a self-limited illness.

At her first follow-up visit one week later, Mrs. Nash continued to look reasonably healthy. I reviewed the unremarkable scans of her chest and abdomen, important negatives, since fevers and night sweats can be due to lung cancer, lymphoma, or a hidden infection within the abdomen. "Are your fevers and muscle and joint pain any better with the medication I prescribed?"

"Not really," she answered. "If anything, I feel worse, much worse." There was a long pause. "So…you don't know what's wrong with me," she said finally, clicking her purse shut.

"Not yet," I answered. I was taken aback by her lack of confidence in me. After all, this was only our second office visit. Her persistent fevers were puzzling but I was confident that I would clarify the cause.

She held out her hands. "My fingers are killing me." This time, I was sure that three of the knuckles on the right hand and two on the left hand were swollen. When I asked Mrs. Nash to flex her fingers to the palm, she was unable to make a full fist. The swollen joints in her hands placed her within the realm of rheumatoid arthritis. But how could that be? I had never seen a patient develop RA after experiencing daily fevers, cough, and muscle aches. But as one of my partners once remarked, *if you have a patient with RA with unusual signs and symptoms you've never seen, you probably haven't seen enough rheumatoid arthritis.*

"Could I have rheumatoid arthritis?" Mrs. Nash asked. "Larry told me to ask you if that's the problem."

"The tests I've ordered for rheumatoid arthritis are negative," I replied. "But they're often negative early in the disease. So yes, it's possible that you have rheumatoid arthritis." I felt vaguely embarrassed that her husband was the one to bring up a diagnosis that I make routinely. Unconvinced that Mrs. Nash had rheumatoid arthritis, I pressed on in a different track. "When was the last time you had a mammogram, colonoscopy, or Pap smear?"

She pursed her lips. "Last year my mammogram was fine. It's been twenty years, I don't know, maybe longer, since my last Pap. Colonoscopy? Never. I don't know why you need to..."

"I want to emphasize that when we are considering a diagnosis of rheumatoid arthritis without positive blood tests, I have to consider a host of rheumatoid mimics. Unfortunately, from time to time, we've seen cancer trigger fevers, muscle pain, and joint pain. I'd like to set you up for an outpatient colonoscopy and you need to see Dr. Hanson for an updated Pap and pelvic exam."

"Fine." She stood and buttoned her coat. Clearly, this was a touchy subject. Abruptly, she stopped at the door and reached out to the counter to steady herself. Her face was flushed and soaked in sweat. I laid Mrs. Nash down. Joanne placed a thermometer in her mouth and a damp cloth on her forehead. "I...I don't feel well," she whispered. "It's one of those spells."

I glanced at the thermometer: 104 degrees. "Let me call your husband. I want to admit you."

After office hours, and before hospital rounds, I pulled a dog-eared copy of an article on fevers of unknown origin (FUO's) by Drs. Petersdorf and Beeson from my files. Published in 1961, the authors reviewed 100 perplexing cases in which the persistent fevers defied a simple explanation. Arriving at the correct diagnosis requires breadth of knowledge, diligence, skilled consultants, and sometimes, a dash of luck. I knew that even with today's improved technology, FUOs remain a clinical challenge. I'll need some help with this case.

On day one, intravenous antibiotics were started on the recommendation of the infectious disease consultant. Testing for a host of uncommon infections was ordered and came back negative. The fact that I had ordered tests for syphilis and HIV was met with steely-eyed, barely suppressed anger by Mrs. Nash. I wasn't going to engage her in a discussion, saying only that the tests were recommended and were a standard part of the workup for an FUO.

Needless to say, the other studies were normal as well. After four days of persistent fevers and no evidence for infection, infectious disease recommended that I discontinue the antibiotics, and signed off Mrs. Nash's case with the standard, *Thank you for this interesting consultation. Please recontact me if there are new developments.*

I scowled at the note, thinking, *Thank you for abandoning ship*.

Following her discharge, and still spiking fevers, I sent Mrs. Nash south for a second opinion at the Massachusetts General Hospital in Boston. The consulting rheumatologist suggested—but was not absolutely sure—that Mrs. Nash suffered from adult-onset Still's disease. Like so many rare disorders in rheumatology, there is no single conclusive test to confirm adult-onset Still's disease. Her daily fevers and intense muscle and joint pain certainly fit the bill, as did the dramatically elevated inflammatory markers. But patients with Still's disease also develop a transient salmon-colored rash with the nightly fevers, which Mrs. Nash lacked. The rash is so distinctive, it's called a Still's rash. Without the rash, the diagnosis of Still's disease was an expert opinion, not a definitive diagnosis.

At the end of the visit, the Massachusetts General Hospital consultant had recommended a trial of prednisone, to which Mrs. Nash replied: "So, you're going to give me prednisone for a diagnosis you're unsure of, for a duration you can't predict, with side effects worse than the disease?"

"No," the rheumatologist answered, meeting her eyes. "Still's disease can be fatal. If you were my mother, I would suggest a trial of prednisone."

Mrs. Nash was unmoved.

Several months later, I was notified that Mrs. Nash had been admitted again through the emergency room with her unexplained fevers, joint inflammation, and generalized weakness. Before driving to the hospital, I sat quietly at my desk. What was I missing? I pulled out a clean white sheet of paper, and at the top wrote FUO. Beneath this, I subdivided the possible causes into five broad subcategories: Psychiatric, Infection, Connective Tissue Diseases, Malignancy, and Miscellaneous.

Psychiatric? Factitious fevers have always held a notable place in mysterious illnesses. While prim, elderly women are not immune to serious psychopathology (see Arsenic and Old Lace), I'd seen several of Mrs. Nash's spells, and there was nothing to suggest fakery. On the other hand, my mind drifted back to a case of psychogenic FUO in a woman one of my partners consulted on who was admitted with fevers and crops of pustular lesions on the forearms. Despite an extensive workup, the daily fevers persisted and new lesions erupted.

After cultures of the mysterious boils and a biopsy of the skin was inconclusive, a simple explanation ensued. A food service worker accidentally bumped the patient's purse off the edge of the bed and spilled a dozen filthy needles filled with a mysterious brown substance onto the floor. The patient was confronted and left the hospital against medical advice before psychiatry could evaluate her.

Had I fully ruled out infection? It is difficult to prove a negative. The usual suspects had been ruled out. I recalled that the Chikungunya virus, found primarily in Africa and a cause of fevers and incapacitating muscle and joint inflammation, had recently been reported in the southern United States. I flipped back to the infectious disease consult. Mrs. Nash and her husband had vacationed in Florida the week before they became ill. I wrote down Chikungunya, knowing full well that the virus was not listed as a cause of chronic fevers. This was a rheumatologic Hail Mary.

Under connective tissue diseases, I felt confident I had ruled out lupus and a host of other rare disorders, but the Massachusetts General rheumatologist's possible diagnosis of adult-onset Still's disease remained a possibility. Because the characteristic rash of Still's disease may appear only with evening fevers, I wrote: *Visit patient in evening to look for Still's rash*, and circled my comment in red.

Malignancy? I reconsidered the original hematology opinion. It came early in the workup when the hematologist considered Mrs. Nash's mild anemia to be secondary to intense inflammation. On the other hand, we were months into her illness, the anemia was worse, and I had imaged nearly every nook and cranny of her body. I wrote: *bone marrow aspiration and biopsy?* And circled it, twice.

Beneath miscellaneous, I wrote: *unusual case of sarcoidosis?* I'd seen a handful of patients with this mysterious inflammatory illness over the years, but the diagnosis was made by sampling an enlarged lymph node in the chest or abdomen. There were no enlarged lymph nodes in Mrs. Nash's chest or abdomen. Nevertheless, I circled sarcoidosis and allowed it to remain.

I folded up the single page and placed it inside my pocket calendar. Before leaving for the hospital, I skimmed through a newly published article on fevers of unknown origin. In the summary, I noticed something I'd overlooked in my previous readings: In all of the FUO published reports, whether the patient was evaluated at the Mayo Clinic, a community hospital in Maine, or Guy's Hospital in London, anywhere from 5-15% of those afflicted by FUO remained an enigma. For a small subset of patients, there simply was no explanation for their illness.

When I walked into Mrs. Nash's room that evening with the family practice resident, Dr. Nash reached up and wiped his eyes with the back of his hand. In his years as a surgeon, I'm sure he had seen his share of tough, hopeless cases. But those patients had a terminal diagnosis; they were dying from inoperable cancer or tragic accidents. Over the last four months, as he watched his wife suffer, he'd transitioned to a full-time caregiver, with no clear answers in sight. He met my eyes and shrugged.

"I'm so tired," Mrs. Nash whispered almost inaudibly. "Am I dying?" I sat down on the edge of her bed. Her nurse recorded a temperature of 103.8 and entered the data into the bedside computer. Then, Dr. Nash did a lovely thing. He reached over and gently massaged his wife's neck and shoulders. She relaxed. We all relaxed.

From my shirt pocket, I retrieved my cheat sheet of differential diagnosis, my Rosetta Stone of diagnostic possibilities. "I have a few ideas," I said, more confidently than I felt. "I've called hematology. Dr. Ebrahim has set aside time tomorrow morning to perform a bone marrow biopsy. We'll be drawing more blood for additional testing. For now, [What was this, the fourth time I'd suggested steroids?] I want to start an intravenous dose of prednisone." I paused. "It's time. I think it will help."

"Okay." Her eyes remained half-closed. "But not too high a dose." Another moment of silence. "Okay, whatever you think I need."

Within hours of the first dose, Mrs. Nash's fever resolved, and she slept through the night for the first time in months. By morning, Mrs. Nash's joints were remarkably improved, but the cause of her illness remained a mystery. She paced the hallway in preparation for her upcoming bone marrow biopsy, not out of worry, but with excess energy—a common side effect of prednisone. Her nurse reported that Mrs. Nash had one remaining complaint; she had critiqued the quality of her breakfast and found it substandard. This boded well for an early discharge.

Dr. Ebrahim, the hematologist, stopped by after breakfast, and after positioning Mrs. Nash on her side, opened his bone marrow procedure tray, anesthetized the skin and deeper tissues with an injection of lidocaine, and expertly removed a plug of bone from her pelvic bone. He followed this by aspirating a sample of bone marrow cells, apologized for the discomfort, and quietly left the room. When the pathologist called me that afternoon, I was fully prepared for a normal result. But this time, there *was* an answer: Clusters of inflammatory cells were scattered throughout the specimen.

"There's no sign of cancer?"

"No signs of cancer."

"Are the inflammatory cells suggestive of sarcoidosis?" I asked cautiously.

"Yes. The biopsy is absolutely consistent with sarcoidosis. As you know, it's unusual for sarcoidosis to be confined to the bone marrow. I reviewed her chart and apparently it hasn't shown up anywhere else."

I ran my hand through my hair before answering. "Well, it's been a long road, but sarcoidosis can be an elusive diagnosis. I'm good with that. Thanks."

Hanging up, I recalled another case of sarcoidosis from when I was an internal medicine resident. I'd presented the findings of a newly admitted patient with daily fevers, cough, and painful ankle swelling to Phil Slocum, DO, my attending physician. When I had finished, he hung her chest X-ray on the view box and said, "Good summary. Now the hard part. Tell me what you think is wrong with this patient."

Instead of answering directly, I felt my way along, sorting the evidence. "Our patient has warm, swollen ankles and her laboratory studies show intense inflammation. The lymph nodes on the chest X-ray adjacent to the heart are enlarged. The lymph nodes could be related to an infection, and of course we should add malignancy to the list, but with the ankle inflammation, I believe it's more likely the patient has sarcoidosis. We should arrange for a biopsy of one of the lymph nodes."

"Are you sure?" Dr. Slocum asked.

"Of the diagnosis of sarcoidosis? No. It's a rare disease. I've never seen it before. But I'm certain that we should consider the diagnosis and obtain a biopsy."

"Excellent," Slocum replied. "Most excellent. Even a blind pig will find an acorn now and then."

Twenty years later, Mrs. Nash's bone marrow biopsy had confirmed another diagnosis of sarcoidosis. I had found another acorn.

Postscript

During the next year, each time I tried to slowly taper Mrs. Nash's daily prednisone, her fevers and joint inflammation relapsed. On the prednisone, she gained weight, transitioned into full-blown diabetes, and developed osteoporosis. These were not pleasant visits.

Fortunately, she agreed to a second medication, a biologic response modifier called adalimumab, with the hope that it would allow her to eliminate daily prednisone. Six months later she took her last dose of prednisone and remains in remission on the new medication. Several years ago, she celebrated her 50th anniversary.

Chapter 19

"No matter how much falls on us, we keep plowing ahead.
That's the only way to keep the roads clear."
Greg Kincaid

A raw, ground-hugging mist enveloped the golf course. Eighteen-year-old Chuck N. led several hundred runners at the two-mile mark at the Maine State High School Cross-Country Championships. Heavily favored to win the race, he faded in the last mile but managed to hang on to eleventh place, with four of his teammates following immediately behind to narrowly claim the team title. Looking back now, his mother remembers her concern when he collapsed to the ground, and how long he remained there, his chest heaving, while his teammates piled on top celebrating the victory. When he hugged her afterwards, his fingers felt stone-cold. It was the first time that she noticed the blanching in several of his fingers.

Several days later, his mother and father were disappointed when, without explanation, Chuck bailed on a family hike up Mount Washington they had planned for months. Their son had always been self-contained, guided by his own inner compass, driven, actually. They wondered whether losing the race was more of a disappointment than he let on. They gave him space.

A month after the championship race, Chuck still felt exhausted and weak. Each morning, after washing up, he returned to his bedroom, stretched and began his routine. First squats, then pushups. In preparation for his senior year, the previous summer he had worked his way up to 100 push-ups and 300 sit-ups. Now, the muscles in his thighs trembled when he tried to complete a set of 10 simple squats. When his girlfriend noticed that he was breathing hard hurrying to a class, she wondered if he had developed asthma.

The last time he was able to run, snow gently fell on his favorite trail in a nearby park. He jogged—barely faster than a brisk walk—as the path zigzagged through a stand of red spruce up a gentle incline. Lightheaded, he stopped and felt for his pulse. It took ten minutes for his heart rate and breathing to return to baseline. Then he followed his tracks slowly home in the snow.

On Christmas Eve, when his mother watched her son struggle to climb the two flights of stairs to the family's duplex, he was secretly relieved and agreed that it was time to see a doctor.

Dr. Rand, who had known the family since they had moved to town 15 years before, was shocked to hear faint crackles in the bottom third of each lung. On a hunch, when he tested Chuck N.'s strength in the shoulders and thighs, he found subtle but definite weakness, a surprising finding in an 18-year-old. Dr. Rand excused himself and called my rheumatology practice. I was on call that week and agreed to see Chuck that afternoon.

By the time I settled into a chair inside the exam room with Chuck and his parents, I'd reviewed the results of his chest X-ray and preliminary tests that had been faxed to my office. I scribbled down notes and fleshed out the timeline of Chuck's illness, aware of the concept of the "magic minute," the first minute of an encounter when clinicians should listen to the patient's story without interruptions or distractions. Doing so not only provides important clues to diagnosis, but helps establish trust. When this has been measured in research studies, the results have been disappointing; the patient's opening statement typically lasts 40 seconds, but physicians tend to interrupt after about 20 seconds.

At six-foot-two, Chuck had the presence of an elite distance runner: long-legged, sinewy, and barrel-chested. A recent attempt at a scraggly beard—it was coming in in shades of copper and blond masked a faint, crimson discoloration on the cheeks. The eyelids were slightly swollen with a hint of violet. Over the knuckles of the hands was another slightly raised rash called Gottron's papules. Together, the signs suggested dermatomyositis (DM), an autoimmune disease with an uncertain prognosis.

How specific are the rashes of dermatomyositis? I like to think that if I noticed them on a stranger in the checkout line at a grocery store, I would introduce myself, discretely inquire if the rash was new and ask if they had noticed any weakness. Of course, the reality of my musings, the more likely scenario, is that I would have been embarrassed, allowed the moment to pass, and wondered if I could have facilitated an important diagnosis.

I reconfirmed Dr. Rand's findings of subtle weakness in the muscles of the shoulders and thighs with normal strength in his grip and lower legs. But it was Chuck's lung exam that was most disconcerting. The prominent crackles in both lower lung fields were suspicious for interstitial lung disease (ILD), inflammation of the connective tissue between the smallest airways and delicate capillaries of the lung where oxygen and carbon dioxide are exchanged. Not all dermatomyositis patients develop ILD, but the finding dispelled any lingering doubt that the disease was limited to the skin and muscles and placed Chuck in a category of extreme concern. Where else might the inflammation be smoldering?

Joanne knocked on the door and handed me the results of the blood work from Dr. Rand's office. The CPK testing, a measurement of muscle inflammation, showed a level of 3,100—more than 15 times the upper limit of normal, and indicated severe muscle inflammation. After completing the exam, I turned my chair towards Chuck and addressed him directly; after all, at 18 he was technically an adult. His parents seemed comfortable holding their questions until I had answered Chuck's.

"Dermatomyositis—we often shorten the name to DM—is a rare condition," I began. "Although we suspect that the disease may sometimes be triggered by a virus, in most cases the cause remains unknown. What we *do know* is that the immune system in DM becomes misdirected, triggering inflammation both in the skin and muscles of the shoulders and thighs. The inflammation leads to weakness in the affected muscles. In some cases, and I suspect this has happened to you, the inflammation can also affect the lungs, which is why you're short of breath when you climb stairs or try to run."

I paused. Chuck scratched his chin and looked at me directly. "Okay. I get that. I overheard Dr. Rand tell my parents that he suspected dermatomyositis, so I checked it out online. A lot of it I don't understand. It's like doctors speak a foreign language. But I get the basics: my immune system is screwed up, nobody understands exactly what went wrong, and I can't run anymore. What do I take to make it go away?"

I am thinking: *mature, direct, confident.* "Good question. Treating dermatomyositis will require intensive treatment with more than one drug to suppress the inflammation, and I'm sorry to tell you this, Chuck, but this won't be like a course of antibiotics; you'll need to take these medications for many months, and your progress will be slow."

"How soon will I run again?"

I hedged. Doctors are terrible at predictions. "It may be many months. There's tremendous variation in how this disease responds to medications. I'm sorry I can't be more specific. Our first goal is to stop your decline." Pausing, I changed the subject. "I'm going to arrange for you to see several other doctors this week who will help us clarify the extent and severity of your disease. Similar to your cross-country team, we need a strong medical team to develop a successful game plan."

I turned to Chuck's parents. "I'll make arrangements with Dr. Slocum, a lung specialist, to see your son this week. We also need a biopsy of the thigh muscle to confirm the diagnosis of dermatomyositis. We'll get that scheduled as soon as possible through one of the general surgeons. As soon as the muscle biopsy is performed, we'll begin treatment with a medication called prednisone." The parents were familiar with prednisone. It turned around a nasty case of poison ivy Chuck acquired on a family camping trip. His mother, an elite distance runner in high school and college, had taken it several times for flares of asthma.

On a hunch, I excused myself from the room and brought back a pulse oxygen saturation unit and placed it on Chuck's right index finger. After a few seconds the digital result appeared on the screen: 97% oxygen saturation, the same normal result that Joanne had registered when she had taken his vital signs 20 minutes earlier. Then I asked Chuck to walk briskly down the hallway with me. By the time we returned to the room, Chuck was winded and the oxygen level had dropped to 91%, clearly abnormal. Internally, I was deflated. This was far worse than I had expected.

Chuck's oxygen level after briskly walking roughly 50 feet was similar to an elderly patient with moderately severe emphysema.

I asked Chuck's parents if they had any questions. Shell-shocked, they shook their heads and quietly followed their son to the checkout counter.

For a moment I remained seated in the room, reviewing the visit. The rapid progression of Chuck's breathlessness since his last cross-country race was worrisome. On the other hand, I'd seen patients with similar presentations respond rapidly to treatment. It was too early to make predictions. I needed more data.

I glanced at the clock, pivoted and picked up the chart of my next patient, Amanda N., my sometimes-incorrigible lupus patient, still working for the past six years in a veterinarian practice thirty minutes outside of Portland. Skimming through her chart, I reviewed her last office visit. On a daily dose of Plaquenil, she had been in remission.

Not today. Opening the exam door, I could see at a glance that Amanda's wrists were red and swollen. On her face was a slightly raised butterfly-shaped rash, the wings extending onto both cheeks. She grimaced as she shifted position and sheepishly admitted that she had vacationed recently in Bermuda with her fiancé, Paul, the veterinarian. "I really tried to stay out of the sun, wore lots of sunblock, but...I guess it wasn't enough," she shrugged. "The lab drew my blood on the way in. I hope it's not too screwed up."

I was prepared for, well, anything. Amanda's internal organs often took the brunt of her flares. This time her blood counts and kidney function were surprisingly stable, and I was optimistic that her lupus flare would come under good control by restarting a brief course of prednisone. Years ago, at the word *prednisone,* Amanda's reaction would have been predictable outrage. This time, she took a deep breath before admitting, "I thought you were going to prescribe prednisone today. I mean, it could be worse. Can you keep the dose low?"

"Let's start with 15 mg daily. I'll see you back next week. If a low dose of prednisone isn't sufficient to control your flare, there's a new lupus medication called Benlysta that we can discuss. I don't like prednisone any more than you do."

For the first time, I noticed her engagement ring and the full impact of...*my fiancé, Paul,* finally registered. Amanda engaged? With the onset of her disease at age 12 through her tumultuous, noncompliant teenage years, I was grateful that she wasn't on dialysis, or worse. Engaged? I extended a hand before she pulled me in for a long hug.

After lunch, I called Dr. Slocum, the pulmonologist, and he agreed to see Chuck N. the next day. Out of curiosity, I spoke with our laboratory director and discovered that the specialized panel of tests for dermatomyositis I had ordered would be sent to Pittsburgh's Presbyterian Medical Center, the training site for my rheumatology fellowship. I jotted down in my pocket calendar: *Present case at rheumatology conference next week,* then added: *get gas for boat; remember to get out early for Molly's school play and Kate's indoor track meet this week.*

For three days, nothing, then the muscle biopsy results returned and the preliminary results confirmed the diagnosis of dermatomyositis. Later that day, I received a call from Dr. Slocum, who had performed a bronchoscopy—a procedure where a flexible scope is passed into the lung—and was concerned about the amount of scarring already present on the biopsy.

When I called Chuck's mother with the results, she was relieved that her son would be starting treatment with prednisone. Her voice quivered, "This is just overwhelming. Everything is coming at us way too fast. Chuck seems to be handling this far better than my husband and me." I had no ready answer, no platitude for her distress. I asked her to make a list of questions for their follow-up visit and said we would take as much time as needed to answer them.

Following the phone call, I placed Chuck's chart aside for my weekly rheumatology conference at Maine Medical Center. There, I presented Chuck's case to my partners. The group agreed with my initial treatment with high-dose prednisone. One of the most experienced rheumatologists added, "I don't like the pace of his disease. He's gone from an elite runner to being out of breath with two flights of stairs. Let's just hope that the Pittsburgh lab finds an Mi-2 antibody."

We all shared this hope. The Mi-2 antibody—one of more than a dozen antibodies that can be found in the blood of patients with dermatomyositis—is usually associated with a good treatment response. For some fortunate Mi-2 patients, this means that over the course of a year, there may be a complete recovery, and in some, medications can be discontinued. A week later, the results from the Pittsburgh lab came across my desk, and they couldn't have been worse. A rare antibody called signal recognition protein (SRP) was present, a marker for difficult to treat, sometimes intractable disease.

I emailed one of my former colleagues at the University of Pittsburgh, rheumatologist Chester Oddis, MD, and included the muscle biopsy results and the finding of the SRP antibody. Unexpectedly, an hour later, he e-mailed back. *Tough case. As you know, SRP patients sometimes don't improve with conventional treatment but very unusual to have lung damage this severe so early. If you haven't done so yet, obtain an echocardiogram to ensure that the heart muscle isn't involved. Consider combination therapy with Cytoxan or Rituxan. Perhaps your patient can be in a research study through us?*

I opened my pocket calendar and scribbled: *Pittsburgh consult?*

That evening, as I motored slowly home across the moonless bay with Kate (in track shorts and T-shirt), and Molly (wrapped in a parka but dressed as a dog from her evening play), I recalled Maine author Stephen King's observation: "Life turns on a dime. Sometimes towards us, but more often it spins away, flirting and flashing as it goes..." As I concentrated on the distant lights of Peaks Island, a lobster buoy rolled under the bow and spun harmlessly away from my propeller. I glanced at the gas tank. Full. My navigational lights were working. I was several hundred yards south of the exposed ledges off House Island.

From a travel bag, Sandi calmly handed out extra sweatshirts, knit caps, and mittens, eventually satisfied that our children were relatively comfortable for our frigid trip home. When I asked Kate where her sweatpants and mittens were, the ones she wore to school that morning, she shrugged, "I have no idea." Like father, like daughter.

That evening, as I sat steaming away the stress of the day in our sauna, I recalled another young man I had taken care of with dermatomyositis at Pittsburgh's Presbyterian Medical Center. Three years into treatment, his muscle weakness had progressed to the point where he needed a walker to use the bathroom. Prednisone had led to a 50-pound weight gain, diabetes, recurrent infections, and several painful spinal fractures from prednisone-induced osteoporosis.

When he was hospitalized with yet another pneumonia, I stopped by on rounds to assess his progress. Removing his oxygen briefly, he pointed to a Polaroid camera on the bed stand and asked his nurse if she would take a picture of us. Unsaid was his intent; he wanted me to remember him. We both knew that he was in a downward spiral. He had undergone trials with both conventional and experimental medications and none of the medications had touched his disease.

It was the first time that I had treated a dermatomyositis patient with the signal recognition protein (SRP) antibody.

Shortly after moving back to Maine, I learned that he had passed away—at age 32—leaving behind a wife and two sons. From time to time, I've taken out his photo from my files and studied his eyes, weary after years of steady decline. Even to the end, he still held out hope that a new drug would turn his life around.

In my early years of practice, discouraged by my failures, I sometimes pictured my patients pouring into a funnel and flowing through the spout, their autoimmune diseases inadequately controlled, adjusting to a future they could never have imagined. Some of them became disabled. More than a few died. Despite this, and more often than one might predict, there were those who lived their lives with gratitude for what they *were* capable of. From these patients, I've learned that it's possible to endure, sometimes even thrive, with diseases that rob us of our dreams.

Today, I expect that my RA patients will be fully functional decades after the mysterious onset of their disease; that my lupus patients will never need dialysis for kidney failure; that my myositis patients will slowly regain their strength. But even today, the funnel analogy holds. Despite recent advances in medications, some diseases continue to progress like a slow-moving, relentless malignancy.

As I tied off SAKAMO to my float and ascended the iron ladder to the wharf, I worried that Chuck N.'s dermatomyositis would be one such case. His lungs already had taken a direct hit. In cases such as his, what we see on lung scans is always a mixture of scar tissue and inflammation. The inflammation we can treat, but the scarring? You can't reverse permanent tissue damage. Watching his oxygen levels plummet with a brisk 50-foot walk was an indication of just how far we had to go. I wondered, would Chuck ever run again?

The next morning, I asked Joanne to begin the process of obtaining prior approval for Rituxan from Chuck's mother's health insurance plan. My follow-up visit with Chuck was the following week, but I knew that approval of expensive medications like Rituxan (costing more than $40,000 per year) might be delayed, and I wanted to get the intravenous drug onboard as soon as possible.

At follow-up, Chuck was in good spirits. The rash on his eyelids and fingers had faded but not disappeared. Except for mild insomnia, he was tolerating the high-dose prednisone and his CPK (the measurement of muscle inflammation) was modestly lower. But there was reason for concern. The crackles in the lower third of each lung had expanded into the mid-lungs and Chuck's shoulders and thighs remained weak. Checking my notes, I thought it was odd that Chuck wasn't on the schedule to receive his first intravenous infusion of Rituxan.

After I finished his exam, Chuck's mother pulled out a denial letter she had received that day from her insurance company for the Rituxan. With trembling hands, she read off the reason for the denial: *Rituxan is not currently FDA approved for the treatment of dermatomyositis.* "Dr. Radis, are they saying that Rituxan isn't the right medication for Chuck?"

The letter angered me on a number of levels, not the least that the denial implied a level of mismanagement in her son's care. I exhaled slowly and met her eyes. "Rituxan is definitely the right medication for your son. Because the FDA requires large studies to assess safety and effectiveness, and dermatomyositis is a rare condition, there are no FDA approved medications for the disease. Zero. How do we know Rituximab is effective? I rely on expert opinions based on smaller studies published in medical journals to guide therapy. The people who denied Rituxan for Chuck's dermatomyositis are clerks and administrative workers, not physicians. They have a checklist to follow and based on this they sent you a form letter of denial."

I let this sink in for a moment before Chuck said, "So they control my care. That's crazy."

"No. They'd like to think so, but fortunately we have an employee who will resubmit the prior paperwork with a letter from me clarifying the reasons to approve the Rituxan. I'm going to insist on speaking directly with one of their staff physicians. I'm sure we can move forward with the Rituxan soon."

The flow of the visit had been disrupted. Instead of concentrating on Chuck's complex medical needs during a critical office visit, I had to explain the intricacies of health insurance denials, and how physicians have to fight to do the right thing. Refocusing, I placed the oxygen saturation unit on Chuck's finger and repeated our walk down the hallway and back. The oxygen level dropped to 89%, significantly lower than our initial testing.

Again, I only spoke in general terms, that the value was low, and that it was early in treatment. "It's lower. Isn't it?" Chuck locked eyes with me as he took a seat. "I can feel it. I'm more short of breath than two weeks ago." As a cross-country runner, he was attuned to his body, and he could feel it slowly failing.

"With the delay in the Rituxan…" I turned and addressed his parents, "We're altering course. Tomorrow, I'm arranging for three days of outpatient intravenous treatment with high-dose Solu-Medrol, a liquid form of prednisone. And in preparation for the Rituxan infusion and to lower the risk of infection, I want to add a daily antibiotic to his mix of meds." Then, turning my attention back to Chuck, "I know this sounds like something I'd recommend to an elderly patient, but it wouldn't hurt to get a pill box with separate compartments for each day of the week. It's easy to get mixed up with the pills and miss a dose…or take too many."

Chuck scowled, and slumped further into his chair, but then shrugged. "I'll get a pill box. If I'm breathing like an old man, why shouldn't I take pills like an old man?"

I tapped a finger on the table. My uneasiness simmered just below the surface. No matter what the illness, there is always another specialist with more experience in rare autoimmune diseases. Better to arrange a formal second opinion now than wait. I turned to Chuck's parents. "I'd like to set up a consultation either at the Massachusetts General Hospital in Boston, or where I trained at Presbyterian Medical Center in Pittsburgh. If in the coming weeks, the medications suppress the inflammation and Chuck improves, we can always cancel the second opinion." For a moment, there was an uncomfortable silence. It was a lot to absorb. Chuck's father fidgeted in his chair and glumly looked to his wife.

"I have a sister in Pittsburgh," she said finally. "There is a daily direct flight from Portland to Pittsburgh. Who would the consult be with? My sister is a medical social worker and worked at Pitt several years ago."

"The consult will be with Chester Oddis, MD, a rheumatologist who focuses his clinical work and research on autoimmune muscle disease. I've been in contact with him and he's already familiar with Chuck's case. Let's get the consult scheduled."

The following week, more bad news. The health insurance company was playing more games, this time insisting that they had 14 days to *consider* my request for a physician-to-physician appeal. In response, I faxed an angry rebuttal to their delay game, stating that if the patient continued to decline and suffered permanent lung damage due to denial of an appropriate treatment, I would hold them personally responsible. Before signing off, I added that an investigative reporter from the local newspaper would be contacting them shortly if they did not approve Rituxan. In capital letters I wrote: *THERE ARE NO FDA APPROVED DRUGS FOR DERMATOMYOSITIS. RITUXAN IS A NECESSARY MEDICATION.*

My hand was shaking as I signed off on the fax. Then I tried, unsuccessfully, to clear my mind before seeing my next patient.

The fax must have moved rapidly up the denial chain from the clerk to the supervisor to a physician, because three days later, the Rituxan was approved. At the infusion center on the second floor of our office, Chuck promptly received his first infusion, and two weeks later, his second. Over the next four months, Chuck's muscle strength gradually improved but his lung function barely budged.

Chuck and his mother flew to Pittsburgh for the consultation with Dr. Oddis. He agreed with my strategy of Rituxan infusions every six months, but also introduced them to the possibility of Chuck participating in a study with an experimental medication if the Rituxan lost its effectiveness. Over time, I ever so slowly tapered the oral prednisone in hopes of reducing the risk of infection while pinning my hopes on further infusions of Rituxan.

That April, now six months into his illness, as Sebago Lake iced-out and the winter loons on Casco Bay returned to their home lakes to nest, Joanne pulled me from a patient's room for a phone call. Dr. Slocum wanted me to know that Chuck was on his way to the intensive care unit with pneumonia. "He's already received his first dose of antibiotics." There was a long pause on the phone. "This is going to get worse before it gets better."

When I stopped by the hospital that evening, Chuck lay in a drug-induced coma on a ventilator. Still reasonably fit and healthy appearing, he looked like he might awaken at any moment, pull out the tube and ask if it was okay if he went for a jog. The ICU nurse chatted to him cheerfully—one never knows what our comatose patients overhear, and gentle words of optimism may allay fear—as she hung an IV infusion of steroids and adjusted the tape around Chuck's nose holding the endotracheal tube in place.

I found Chuck's parents huddled together in the family conference room. Extended family members spilled out into the hallway talking quietly, sipping coffee or whispering into their cell phones. Chuck's mother looked up as I entered. I pointed towards a side room where we could have some privacy and took a seat facing the parents with a coffee table between us.

Chuck's mother asked, "Do you have a copy of our last visit with Dr. Oddis?"

"No. Not yet."

She opened her purse and handed me an envelope. "Last week, he mentioned that Chuck's lungs were so scarred that an infection could send him over the edge." She glanced over to her husband and he placed an arm around her shoulder. Her voice dropped to a whisper. "The morning before our flight home, he arranged for us to meet with the lung transplant team. After our meeting with the doctors, they presented Chuck's case at their weekly conference and…" her voice cracked, "Chuck is on the double-lung transplant list."

I was not surprised. Presbyterian Medical Center was a leader in transplantation medicine. Thomas Starzl, MD, pioneered the world's first successful liver transplant there, and had subsequently trained a generation of skilled surgeons now performing transplants in major medical centers in the United States and around the world. Chuck would be in good hands.

On his fourth day on the ventilator, Chuck had improved enough that the ICU medical team discontinued his sedation, and he began to communicate via pen and paper. What did he want? He requested weights to strengthen his arms and legs. Under the direction of a physical therapist (to avoid entangling his IV lines) he broke out in a heavy sweat as he strained to complete three sets with the ten-pound weights. Exhausted, he drifted off to sleep.

One week later, Chuck was weaned off the ventilator and moved to the general floor. By then, he had resumed his deep knee bends and independent weight lifting. This was a challenge he understood. He was back in training, setting new goals as he met his own standards of recovery. But there were limits. Prior to his hospitalization, he had worn the oxygen only while exercising; now, he required it day and night.

But he stayed on the list.

That fall, instead of attending college, Chuck was hired as an assistant coach in cross-country for his former high school team. At practice, he wore a mask to lower the likelihood of developing another pneumonia and met with the team outside, wearing his portable oxygen tank on a shoulder strap. After cross-country season, as he rose higher on the transplant list, his mother took a leave of absence from work and the two moved temporarily to Pittsburgh to stay with her sister while they awaited word from the transplant coordinator. His father remained in Maine with the couple's junior high daughter.

Then early one predawn November morning, I received a text from his mother in Pittsburgh: *Chuck is in surgery for two new lungs. Wish us luck.* I looked in on my sleeping daughters, kissed Sandi goodbye, and walked up to the truck. Someone, I knew, had to die so that Chuck could live. Motorcycle accident? Aneurysm dissection? Brain tumor?

The keys were next to the stick shift. I felt in my pocket for my wallet. Check. Cell phone? Check. Hearing aids? Check. Sandi opened our front door, dangling my boat keys in her hand, and proceeded up the walkway wrapped in a light burgundy parka, her breath misting overhead, her slippers leaving a sharp outline in the frost. When she reached the truck, I was sobbing. It had been a long time since I'd cried. She stood next to the truck, her hand on my shoulder through the open window. "News from the hospital?"

"Transplant kid. He's getting a new set of lungs in Pittsburgh."

"Well, he's in good hands. I'm sure it's going to go well."

On my drive to the dock, I passed by the Peaks Island Health Center (where I practiced primary care medicine more than 20 years ago), and recognized the cottage of Lois H. A smile slowly stretched across my face as I recalled a visit with her at the health center in the midst of a raging snowstorm.

All of my patients had canceled their appointments that morning, and I was alone at the clinic doing paperwork when I heard a knock on the door. Lois trudged in and took a seat. For an older woman who took great pride in her appearance, she looked like she'd been out all night on a bender. I asked what was wrong and somewhat sheepishly, she admitted that on the way to the bathroom the previous evening, she had tripped on a rug, stumbled across the living room, and fell backwards into a lobster trap she used as a magazine stand. The glass top shattered and she came to rest with her rearend and back wedged into the lobster trap. She couldn't move. "I was trapped by the trap!" A neighbor heard her cries for help the next morning, and extricated Lois from her predicament with the aid of a handsaw. "Frankly, I'm relieved that the rescue squad wasn't called. My dress was up over my head. I looked like an upside-down turtle."

After her back fracture healed, Lois lived another 10 years before she died at age 89.

At the pier, I climbed down the iron-rung ladder, started the engine, and released the lines. On a hunch, I typed into my cell phone: *Can a lung transplant patient run after surgery?* I clicked on a connecting website and learned that, *yes, lung transplant patients have even run a marathon.* My mind settled. Sandi was right when she predicted, "I'm sure it's going to go well." Lois and Chuck were cut from the same cloth. In Finland, they call it *sisu*, a melding of resilience, grit, tenacity, and perseverance.

Midway across the harbor, the sun rose over Peaks Island. A flock of cormorants dove into a school of baitfish off Fort Gorges. Two harbor porpoises plunged repeatedly into the school, then rocketed from the water chasing the fleeing fish. I cut the engine and drained the last of my morning coffee. In another moment, the water settled, the porpoises scattered, and the cormorants, their wings skimming the surface, flew off towards deeper water.

I pulled out my office schedule and ran a finger down the list. Some of my patients, hopefully most, will be doing well. Some, inevitably, will not be well. I circled the names of my three new consults. I'll hear their stories, weigh the evidence, and hopefully come up with a diagnosis and plan of treatment. It's time to get to work.

Acknowledgements

Like many physicians, my road to medical school was not a straight line. Before my father died when I was eleven, there was stability, parental guidance, and structure. Afterwards, although my mother tried in vain to rein in my recklessness and impulsiveness, I would have gone off the rails if not for my lifelong connection to my childhood friends. Raise a glass to my neighborhood pals: Tux Turkel, Bruce Hogan, Rob Mintz, Rich Ferdinand, Martin Kane, George Backinoff, Jeff Freeman, and Bob Rudolph. Your friendship continues to burn bright.

Thank you to the professors and physicians who influenced me at pivotal points in my life, particularly Andrew Balber, PhD, an immunology professor at Bates College, and Lawrence Newth, DO, and Edward Stiles, DO, who encouraged me to apply to osteopathic medical schools.

Phil Slocum, DO, you ran a tight ship as the Director of the Internal Medicine Residency at the small community hospital where I trained. Your reliance on the Socratic method of learning suited me well and I prospered under your tutelage. Your friendship means a lot to me. Paulding Phelps, MD, I am grateful that you encouraged me to apply to a rheumatology fellowship at the University of Pittsburgh. I suspect you played a hand (more than I will ever know) in Thomas Medsger Jr., MD, accepting me as the first DO fellow in the rheumatology department. Thanks also for donating your sauna stove to me so that my Finnish wife, Sandi, can have a proper steam bath.

To the faculty at the University of Pittsburgh: Thomas Medsger Jr., MD, Virginia Steene, MD, Chester Oddis, MD, Kent

Kwoh, MD, Mary Chester Morgan, MD, and many others, the environment you created was inspiring. Patients at the University of Pittsburgh benefited through your spirit of collaboration and deep commitment to patient care.

To my former partners at Rheumatology Associates: Larry Anderson, MD, George Morton, MD, Brian Keroack, MD, Brian Daikh, MD, Stephanie Gartner, MD, and Ed Fels, MD, you demonstrated day in and day out that the practice of rheumatology can excel outside of academic university medical centers. To Geoff Gratwick, MD, and Sid Block, MD, your commitment to serving patients from rural, underserved areas of Maine helped make their journey a little easier.

Thank you also to Steve Landgon for your guidance and editorial help on the manuscript and to my friend Jim McCarthy for designing the cover of *The Mystery in the Room.*

Lastly, my love and heartfelt thanks go to Sandi, my wife of nearly 50 years, and my children, Kate Radis Crothers and Molly Blackburn, and their children: Fiona, Frank, Jett, and Hazel. Over the years, when I've had difficulty saying NO to outside requests and responsibilities, I am gratefully reminded that family comes first. Sandi, you are the glue that holds us all together.

Notes on Sources

Chapter 1

3 Ed Fels, MD, a pediatric rheumatologist, joined Rheumatology Associates in 2009 and continues to provide critically needed care to Maine children, some of whom live more than four hours north of Portland.

12 The information on Plaquenil is taken from a previously published essay of mine, Radis C. (2015). Plaquenil: From Malaria Treatment to Managing Lupus. *The Rheumatologist*, 9(5).

12 Dr. Petri is a strong advocate for avoiding prednisone whenever possible in the management of lupus. It is Dr. Petri who once said, "The P in prednisone stands for poison," a pointed reference to the side effects of prednisone when it is continued long-term. I strive to follow Dr. Petri's advice, but eliminating the use of prednisone completely is not always possible. Dao, K.H. (Nov, 2019). The "P" in Prednisone stands for Poison…and Other Pearls. *Rheum Now Podcast*.

Chapter 2

19 The connection between my father and Rachel Carson and the *Silent Spring* debate on CBS TV, was shared with me by my oldest brother for the first time in 2020, more than 55 years after it occurred. I have no independent

verification of whether this is, in fact, a true story, but as family lore, it has pulled the two of us into a deeper long-term commitment to conservation and love of the outdoors.

23 Dr. Dave was my first connection to the osteopathic profession. In recent years, the number of osteopathic physicians continues to grow. "As of 2024, there were 43 osteopathic medical schools in 36 states. The growth of DO degree-granting institutions has been faster than that of MD medical schools, such that currently 28% of all students pursuing their American medical degrees are enrolled in colleges of osteopathic medicine." Mazzolini C., (2023). The Changing Face of Physicians: The Growth of Osteopathic Medicine, *Medical Economics,* 100(10).

Chapter 4

38 The conversations between Dr. Medsger and myself (like a number of conversations which take place in *The Mystery in the Room*), did not occur as written. As narrative nonfiction, they capture Dr. Medsger's high expectations for his fellows, his critical analysis of clinical information, and his gentle way of dealing with patients with the dreadful disease scleroderma.

46 Rodnan, G.P, and Benedek, T. (1962). An Historical Account of the Study of Progressive Systemic Sclerosis (Diffuse Scleroderma), Annals of Internal Medicine, 57(2), 305-319.

Chapter 5

56 Although Maine is a sparsely populated rural state, there have been a surprising number of remarkable rheumatologists who have practiced here. At age 35, Currier McEwen, MD, became Dean of the School of Medicine at New York University. In 1939 he partnered with Albert Einstein to resettle Jewish doctors and scientists from Nazi Europe in the United States. He retired to Maine at age 68 but due to a shortage of rheumatologists, continued to staff rural clinics in northern Maine until he fully retired from medicine at age 82. Dr. McEwen was a world-renowned hybridizer of Japanese and Siberian iris. He lived in Harpswell, Maine, until he died in 2003 at age 101. His hybridizing efforts resulted in the introduction of over 160 iris cultivars. Ferrell, K., and Brasington, R. (2016). Currier McEwen, MD, Remembered as Rheumatologist, Hybridizer of Flowers, *The Rheumatologist,* 10(3).

57 Dr. Larry Anderson and Dr. Sid Block have been recognized as Master Rheumatologists by the American College of Rheumatology. In his spare time, Larry Anderson managed a tree farm. Block cofounded a Jewish synagogue in Bangor, Maine, and became cantor despite an inability to read music. He retired from his rheumatology practice at age 80. Block's medical partner, Dr. Geoffrey Gratwick, while continuing to practice rheumatology, successfully ran for a seat in the Maine State Senate after a stint as mayor of Bangor.

Chapter 6

65 This chapter on a patient with Whipple's disease is adapted from a previously published article of mine, Radis, C., (2015). The Rheumatologist as Detective: How to Read the Clues to Find the Diagnosis, The Rheumatologist, 9(2), 1, 23-33.

Chapter 7

90 The term granulomatosis with polyangiitis is a recent construct and officially replaced the original eponym, Wegener's granulomatosis in 2010. Although Friedrich Wegener was the first to comprehensively describe the disease which later bore his name, he had extensive ties to Nazism. This change by the American College of Rheumatology reflects ongoing concern with naming and honoring diseases after their discoverer. Arkuszewski, P., Cieslak-Arkuszewska, (2025). Undisclosed Facts in Friedrich Wegener's Links with Nazism; *Histopathology*, 86(3):317-32.

Chapter 8

102 In the March 2012 issue of *The Atlantic* magazine, Teju Cole, a Nigerian American writer, described western overseas volunteer medical missions as: "Medical missions are about a big emotional experience that

validates privilege… If we are going to interfere in the lives of others, a little due diligence is a minimum requirement."

I own my own discomfort and guilt associated with my early forays into medical mission work. These clinics in Ghana and Guatemala were characterized by long lines of patients who received cursory examinations, short-term sample medications, and little, if any, follow-up. Although the volunteer physicians, nurses, and medical students returned to the United States with a glow of self-satisfaction, in my mind, the work should have been focused on more lasting collaborative public health projects. Indeed, in recent years, more emphasis *is* being placed on connecting with local medical practitioners and funding public health initiatives. But even in these projects, there can be an element of White Savior pride if projects are not developed hand-in-hand with local populations. For instance, non-profit western organizations frequently develop clean water projects by digging wells. If the well breaks down, the long-term success of these projects should be measured by whether local technicians have received adequate training and tools to facilitate repairs.

Chapter 9

112 In 1949, Philip S. Hench presented his research findings on the isolation of a remarkable extract from the human adrenal gland he called substance E to an enthusiastic audience of physicians at the International Congress of Rheumatic Diseases. Treatment with substance E resulted

in dramatic improvement in patients with long-standing rheumatoid arthritis. The lecture was "... greeted by the hundreds of attendees with thunderous applause and shouting, with many physicians rushing on the stage to congratulate and embrace Hench..." In the ensuing weeks and months, the side effects of cortisone (prednisone is a synthetic derivative of Hench's original substance E) became woefully apparent. Higher and higher doses were necessary to maintain improvement and patients developed brittle bones, diabetes, and frequent infections. Physicians in every specialty continue to balance the dramatic effectiveness of prednisone verses its dangerous side effects associated with long-term use. Matteson, E.L., Hunder, G. (2024). Philip S. Hench and the Discovery of Cortisone. *Annals of the Rheumatic Diseases*, (83)6, 700-705.

Chapter 10

123 Although my panic attacks were not directly related to the pressures of clinical work, Susan Koven, MD, writes in her chapter of, *Masterclass in Medicine: Lessons from the experts*, (2025) p. 22-30, that "mental illness is common in physicians with high rates of burnout, alcoholism and addiction, and suicide (especially women). A startling 2019 study revealed that 40% of female physicians start practicing part-time or leave clinical medicine altogether within six years of completing residency."

Chapter 11

127 Gold treatment for rheumatoid arthritis dates back to the pre-antibiotic era when the disease was thought by some physicians to be a variant of tuberculosis and heavy metals such as gold injections were often administered. Surprisingly, in some patients, gold was an effective therapy for their RA (about 20% went into a long-term remission while receiving gold injections). In recent decades, much safer and effective treatments have been developed and the goals treatment goals, no pain or swelling, full function, and no X-ray evidence of disease progression, are now frequently met.

Chapter 12

130 This chapter on the possible connection between autoimmune diseases and silicone breast implants is adapted from a previously published article of mine, Radis, C., (2018). Scleroderma: A Case Based Clinical Review, *The Rheumatologist*; 12(2), 1,68-71.

Chapter 13

148 In my own clinical practice, the number of patients who dutifully follow a low-purine diet is extraordinarily low. On the other hand, many of my gout patients are able to

adopt a Mediterranean diet based on fruits, vegetables, whole grains, nuts, seeds, and fish (and little or no alcohol). The Mediterranean diet also reduces the risk of both diabetes and heart disease, and may help in weight control.

Chapter 14

164 The issue of individual and corporate responsibility in the narcotic epidemic has slowly played out in the courts. A few executives have gone to jail. John N. Kapoor, the founder of Insys Therapeutics, was sentenced to 66 months in prison for bribing doctors to prescribe a nasal spray formulation of the highly addictive drug fentanyl. Alec Burlakoff, the former vice president of sales at Insys Therapeutics, pleaded guilty to racketeering and received a 26-month prison sentence. Laurence Doug III at Rochester Drug Cooperative, was sentenced to 27 months in prison for conspiring to unlawfully distribute controlled substances. Lawsuits against Purdue Pharma and other narcotic manufacturers have made their way through the court system. The latest settlement was approved by a federal judge in June 2025. Pending a final vote on the settlement, victims and state and local governments will receive a total of $7.4 billion (which includes contributions from Purdue Pharma and the Sackler family, its former owners). No members of the Sackler family have gone to jail.

Chapter 15

170 In my early years practicing rheumatology, roughly fifteen per cent of my consultations and follow-up office visits were with patients with fibromyalgia syndrome. A medical student rotating in my office, Judith Ziegler, DO, was shocked by how many of my "refractory" fibromyalgia patients had histories of adverse childhood or adult experiences, including physical and sexual abuse, severe car accidents, or other near-death experiences. At the time, the connection between these events and an increased incidence of chronic pain, including fibromyalgia syndrome, was not generally accepted. In recent years, a number of studies have documented higher rates of chronic pain in patients experiencing these life events. In these patients, cognitive behavioral therapy and "mind-body" practices such as tai chi and yoga hold great promise in helping patients better manage their chronic pain. Bacon, A.M., White, L., (2022). The Association Between Adverse Childhood Experiences, Self-Silencing Behaviors and Symptoms in Women with Fibromyalgia. *Psychology, Health & Medicine,* (28) 8, 2073-2083.

174 Canadian physician Harvey Moldofsky was one of the first researchers to link chronic, fragmented, non-restorative sleep to symptoms of fibromyalgia syndrome. Moldofsky, H., Scarisbrick, P., England, H., Smythe, H., (1975). Musculoskeletal Symptoms and non-REM Sleep

Disturbance in Patients with "Fibrositis Syndrome" and Healthy Subjects; *Psychosomatic Med.* 37(4):341-51.

Chapter 16

188 Many studies have documented significant differences in the bowel bacterial biome of patients with active ankylosing spondylitis and patients who are well. Several have documented that the use of biologic treatment with medications such as adalimumab (Humira) can favorably alter this imbalance, but researchers are just beginning to assess whether the use of probiotics can also be an effective treatment tool in patients with active disease. One of the few studies published in The *Journal of Rheumatology* in 2010 did not find significant improvement in disease activity. Jenks, K., et al., (2010). Probiotic Therapy for the Treatment of Spondyloarthritis: a Randomized Controlled Trial, *The Journal of Rheumatology*, (2010) 37(10), 2118-2125.

187 For a full accounting of Muhammad Asim's professional life and artistic gifts, please see: Boonen, A., et al., (2001). Muhammad Asim Khan. Portrait of a Rheumatologist as a Great Artist; *Journal of Rheumatology*, 28(4). 843-844.

Chapter 17

196 This chapter on a patient with psoriatic arthritis who believes he has chronic Lyme disease is adapted from a previously published article of mine, Radis, C., (2016)

The Patient's Choice, When You're the Second (or Third) Opinion. *The Rheumatologist*, 10(2)1, 23-27.

Chapter 18

218 Petersdorf and Beeson's classic article on patients with unexplained fevers remains a helpful starting point in the workup of patients with persistent unexplained fevers. Although more recent reviews demonstrate a changing pattern of diseases and technology has improved, prior to the internet, many physicians kept dog-eared copies of their work in their files to guide the workup of patients with an FUO.

Chapter 19

239 The requirement that healthcare providers seek prior approval for medications or tests is firmly entrenched in the United States medical insurance system. To give an example of how this process delays critically important diagnostic tests and treatment, I would highlight my own former rheumatology practice where we employed a full-time worker whose only job was to submit prior approval requests. On the insurance side, there were employees whose only job was to evaluate (and often deny) requests for prior approval. When the ordering doctor was informed of the denial, he/she would dictate a second request to the insurance company. This back-and-forth process occurred many times each week and led to delays in care. Ultimately, our medical practice almost always overrode denials of care, but the time and money needed

to do right by our patients is one of many reasons why our healthcare system is so expensive and frustrating for both patients and their healthcare providers.

www.ingramcontent.com/pod-product-compliance
Lightning Source LLC
LaVergne TN
LVHW100302210926
848480LV00003B/996